AF614741

CANCER CAUSING SUBSTANCES

Edited by **Faik Atroshi**

Cancer Causing Substances
http://dx.doi.org/10.5772/intechopen.68247
Edited by Faik Atroshi

Contributors

Jian Hai Sun, Zhanwu Ning, Xiaofeng Zhu, Jinhua Liu, Yanni Zhang, Jingjing Zhang, Chunxiu Liu, Trinanjan Basu, Maher Soliman, Vincent Gallicchio, Austin Carver, Michael Higgins, Tara McMorrow, Ismael Obaidi

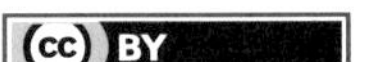

Notice

Statements and opinions expressed in the chapters are these of the individual contributors and not necessarily those of the editors or publisher. No responsibility is accepted for the accuracy of information contained in the published chapters. The publisher assumes no responsibility for any damage or injury to persons or property arising out of the use of any materials, instructions, methods or ideas contained in the book.

First published in London, United Kingdom, 2018 by IntechOpen
IntechOpen is the global imprint of INTECHOPEN LIMITED, registered in England and Wales, registration number: 11086078, The Shard, 25th floor, 32 London Bridge Street
London, SE19SG – United Kingdom
Printed in Croatia

British Library Cataloguing-in-Publication Data
A catalogue record for this book is available from the British Library

Additional hard copies can be obtained from orders@intechopen.com

Cancer Causing Substances, Edited by Faik Atroshi
p. cm.
Print ISBN 978-1-78923-140-3
Online ISBN 978-1-78923-141-0

For EU product safety concerns:
IN TECH d.o.o., Prolaz Marije Krucifikse Kozulić 3, 51000 Rijeka, Croatia,
info@intechopen.com or visit our website at intechopen.com.

Meet the editor

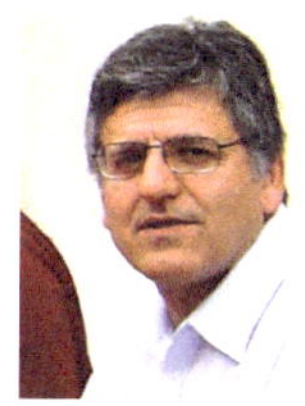

Dr. Faik Atroshi, PhD, is a docent and a senior researcher in Pharmacology and Toxicology at the University of Helsinki, Finland. With a licentiate in biomarkers of health and disease and as an adjunct professor in Clinical Genetics and Nutrition, he is both a senior researcher and a visiting professor in several international institutions and universities, including the Sleep Clinic and Cancer Bio-Immunotherapy Institute, Helsinki, Finland.
He is the director of Education and Research for the Finnish Satellite Center, UNESCO; the president of the International Global Society for Nutrition, Environment, and Health (GSNEH); an editorial board member of the *Scientific World Journal*; and the committee member of the Finnish Medical Physiological Society.

Contents

Preface

The development of cancer is a multistep process in which cells undergo metabolic and behavioral changes, leading to continual unregulated proliferation of cancer cells. Substances that promote carcinogenesis, the formation of cancer, are known as carcinogens. Carcinogens may promote the formation of cancer due to their ability to damage the genome or disruption of cellular metabolic processes. Substances can have different levels of cancer-causing potential; therefore, the risk of developing cancer is dependent on several factors, including individual genetic background and the amount and duration of the exposure.

Consisting of five chapters, this book will examine the impacts of exposure to numerous known, probable, and possible carcinogens in regard to cancer and carcinogenesis. As susceptibility to some of these substances can be notably prevalent in some instances, hopefully, the topic-related review, research, and approaches presented within this book will enable further research as well as development and implementation of beneficial approaches.

The first chapter will examine the concerns regarding exposure to heavy metals, due to the evolving understanding of their role in the development of cancer. This chapter will highlight the research related to the impacts that heavy metals, such as aluminum, arsenic, beryllium, cadmium, lead, mercury, nickel, and radium, have on human health.

The second chapter will examine in detail a number of different aspects of renal cancer with a focus on renal cell carcinomas. This chapter will also take a look at renal cancer from a toxicological point of view along with an in-depth examination of renal carcinogens. This chapter will also examine the different methods currently used to detect a compound's carcinogenic potential.

The third chapter will discuss a growing concern in modern-day society, the current situation of air pollution, and exposure-related cancer risks. This chapter will provide a result-based analysis by presenting the development of a portable environmental gas monitor for rapidly monitoring air pollution, which is able to provide scientific data for environmental pollution control.

The fourth chapter will entail relevant review, research, and findings over selected cancer-causing chemicals and various aspects concerning cancer along with research over mechanisms of carcinogenesis, genotoxic classification, and risk factors associated with substance exposure.

The fifth and final chapter will elaborate on some of the available literature related to two lesser discussed etiologies of cancer, emotional and psychological stress and cell phones, if any links exist between these, and related issues as per different sites of cancers.

Faik Atroshi, PhD, MSc, Lic, Doc
University of Helsinki, Finland

Chapter 1

Heavy Metals and Cancer

Austin Carver and Vincent S. Gallicchio

Additional information is available at the end of the chapter

http://dx.doi.org/10.5772/intechopen.70348

Abstract

There has been increased concern surrounding exposure to heavy metals due to the evolving understanding of their role in the development of cancer. This review highlights research related to the impact that heavy metals aluminum, arsenic, beryllium, cadmium, lead, mercury, nickel and radium have on human health. Research was collected through PubMed, and it was compiled to assess the current knowledge of exposure sources, types of cancers induced and therapeutic measures for these metals. Furthermore, it was designed to assist in guiding future research efforts with respect to heavy metals and cancer.

Keywords: heavy metals, carcinogenesis, exposure, treatment

1. Introduction

Exposure to heavy metals represents significant health concerns in the human population. These elements have the ability to induce a number of adverse health effects, but one of their more serious actions is their role in carcinogenesis. There exists a plethora of information on the research database, PubMed, regarding various exposure patterns and cancers induced by these heavy metals. However, this information has remained largely disconnected at this point, which necessitates the consolidation of this research. Our work reviews studies for how humans are exposed to heavy metals as well as what specific body systems are targeted.

2. Aluminum

Aluminum is a unique heavy metal with numerous pathways of exposure. Exposure to this element has been documented in contaminated food, vaccines to elicit a more powerful immune response and aluminum salts used in industrial processes and commercial products [1, 2].

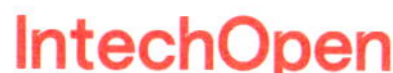

Specific commercial products containing aluminum salts include certain antacids and antiperspirant deodorants [1–3].

Aluminum exposure has been strongly correlated with carcinogenesis in the breast tissue. Mice subjected to $AlCl_3$, the same aluminum salt used in antiperspirant deodorants, displayed malignant growth of mammary gland epithelial cells [1]. This same result was observed in studies performed on samples of human breast cells [1–3]. This heavy metal was also hypothesized to have a role in the development of sarcomas [4]. Additionally, in one patient, it was proposed that the chronic exposure of aluminum containing heavy metal salts resulted in the development of an atypical neuroectodermal tumor [4].

There have been several determined mechanisms for the carcinogenic activity of aluminum. After exposing samples of human breast cells to this element, one study observed diminished concentrations of mRNA for the recognized tumor suppressor gene BRCA1 in addition to mRNA concentrations for other essential DNA maintenance genes [3]. Another study determined that subjecting human breast cells to aluminum had the potential to induce uncontrolled growth [2]. In this study, aluminum was observed to act as a metalloestrogen, which behaves as an agonist for estrogen receptors, and represents a known risk for carcinogenesis in the breast [2]. In another area of the body, analyzed samples of bladder carcinomas displayed statistically higher levels of aluminum, among other heavy metals [5]. Although a mechanism has not been established currently, this evidence suggests that this metal plays at least a supportive role in malignant growth in the bladder [5]. Standard therapy following aluminum poisoning has been the use of chelators. Aluminum in the human body has been demonstrated to bioaccumulate in soft and skeletal tissues, which are target areas for the removal of aluminum [6]. The common chelator used therapeutically has been desferrioxamine [6]. This chelator has proven effective in eliminating aluminum from the body; however, there are a number of toxic side effects associated with its use [6]. There have been several promising candidates to replace desferrioxamine, but none have proved to be as effective thus far [6]. The most successful method in limiting the toxic effects of aluminum is to reduce exposure to the metal. One potential solution for reducing public exposure is the use of reverse osmosis filtration. This technology has demonstrated the ability to remove significant levels of aluminum from copper mining waste at the experimental stage [7].

3. Arsenic

Arsenic is a cytotoxic element, and exposure to this metal presents serious risks to human health. Contact with arsenic generally results from ingesting contaminated food and water, occupational exposure and environmental pollution [8–11] Common occupations where arsenic exposure is common include smelting and arsenic based pesticide industries [12]. One noted source of environmental exposure to this heavy metal is contact with contaminated soil, which has the potential to enter the human food chain [13].

This heavy metal has been detected in an extensive variety of malignant growths. Research strongly supports role of arsenic in the development of lung, bladder and skin cancer [8, 11, 12]. Another study determined a strong positive association between exposure and mortality rates of cancers including colon, gastric, kidney, lung and nasopharyngeal [13]. Epidemiological studies have also suggested an association between chronic low-level exposure to arsenic and development of pancreatic cancer and non-Hodgkin's lymphoma [14, 15].

Well-documented carcinogenic mechanisms for this heavy metal include generation of reactive oxygen species (ROS), epigenetic alterations and damage to the dynamic DNA maintenance system [8, 9, 12]. Key epigenetic changes induced by arsenic include alterations to the status of DNA methylation, histones, and miRNA, which are all changes that have the potential to cause malignant growth [9, 12]. Another study found that this toxic metal could induce inappropriate growth cycles for macrophages in addition to lung epithelial cells [16]. Furthermore, it was observed that macrophages exposed to ROS generated by arsenic responded by activating through the M2 phase, which is correlated with potential lung carcinogenesis [16]. Arsenic displayed a specific mechanism of action against human lung epithelial cells. This heavy metal was determined to alter the expression of the p53 protein, which resulted in decreased expression of p21, one downstream target [17]. The observed inappropriate proliferation was attributed to this mechanism [17]. Further examination of arsenic revealed its ability to reduce intracellular concentrations of glutathione, a natural antioxidant [18]. This carries the potential for carcinogenic activity by subjecting the cell to oxidative stress [18]. An additional carcinogenic mechanism proposed for this heavy metal lies in its ability to influence base excision repair [19]. The enzyme DNA polymerase beta was involved with this repair system, and arsenic was observed to inhibit its activity at high concentrations [19]. Another novel pathway for tumorigenic activity was discovered in human bladder cells. This study determined that chronic arsenic exposure had the potential to induce morphology changes and alter gene expression for proteins that regulate proliferation [20]. The use of chelators has remained the most effective way to eliminate arsenic from the body. Rac-2,3-dimercaptopropanol, or British anti-lewisite, contains two thiol functional groups, and it is one prominent chelator for this metal [21]. Although lacking clinical data at this point, 2,3-dimercaptopropane-1-sulphonate was used in one individual with acute arsenic poisoning [22]. This therapy resulted in successful treatment with limited side effects, which suggests the importance of future study [22]. Following arsenic exposure, dietary antioxidants have been recommended to mitigate carcinogenic effects of this metal, such as oxidative stress [23]. Developing novel prevention methods is essential for limiting human exposure. Rice and apple juice have been recognized as two common sources of exposure [24]. Safety standards of 5 μg/L of arsenic have been recommended for apple juice, due to its extensive ingestion by children [24]. Current research to limit its presence in rice includes genetic modifications to inhibit arsenic uptake, and the use of microbes that compete for arsenic in the environment [24]. It has also been observed that the use of sprinkler irrigation has the potential to significantly reduce the concentration of arsenic in rice by inducing its precipitation [24, 25].

4. Beryllium

Beryllium is a heavy metal that has uses in industrial processes and technology production. The primary environmental contamination source for this element is thought to be power plants, which leech beryllium in the form of dust [26, 27]. Due to inhalation being the general method of exposure for this contaminant, current research is investigating its role in lung carcinogenesis [27–29]. There are mixed reviews supporting the extent of the role for beryllium in lung cancer, but recent research has determined a more significant correlation between the two [28–30]. Furthermore, an increased risk of lung cancer was observed in individuals exposed to exceptionally high concentrations of beryllium, which suggests that this element does induce some carcinogenic mechanism [29]. The use of beryllium in the dental industry creates additional occupational risk for exposure [29]. It was determined that the use of protective equipment significantly reduced the level of exposure in individuals [31]. Additionally, elevated concentrations of beryllium were detected in patients with stage III breast cancer [32]. However, beryllium was one of several heavy metals detected, so a defined role has not been identified at this point [32]. Exposure to beryllium is also recognized as a risk for the potential development of osteosarcomas [33].

Currently, there has not been much research relevant to beryllium's carcinogenic mechanisms. Most literature that exists now is related to action against the lungs. For instance, one potentially carcinogenic mechanism identified was its role in inducing a higher level of tumor necrosis factor alpha (TNF-α) cytokine secretion from CD4+ T-cells in the lungs [30, 34]. Both of these proteins have a role in the inflammation process, and their elevated presence was suspected to have action in chronic inflammation [30, 34]. Beryllium also has the potential to induce inappropriate genetic changes. For instance, this heavy metal was observed to methylate the *p16* gene, a known tumor suppressor gene, and induce its inactivation [30]. Chelators are common forms of therapy used to eliminate beryllium from the body and reduce its toxic effects. Relevant chelators include 4,-dihydroxy-1,3-benzene disulphonic acid disodium salt (Tiron) and D-penicillamine (DPA), which proved to be effective when tested in animals [35–37]. Also, the chelator meso-2,3-dimercaptosuccinic acid (DMSA) was used in a case study to successfully save a child suffering from heavy metal poisoning [38]. This result suggested potential clinical significance and requires further investigation [38]. There have been significant efforts to reduce exposure to this metal, especially occupational exposure [39, 40]. These efforts include company programs instituted to screen blood samples for beryllium sensitization during employment as well as providing refined ventilation and dust control to processes where exposure is common [40]. Attention was also given to educating employees about the importance of using protective equipment, and illuminating the potential risks involved with chronic beryllium exposure [39, 40].

5. Cadmium

Cadmium is an immensely toxic heavy metal, and it is associated with significant health implications as an environmental contaminant. Cadmium contamination generally results from emissions from industries that utilize this element including mining, metal research, development of certain batteries and preventing precipitation in pigments [41]. Soil pollution is a serious issue from cadmium emissions, and human exposure typically occurs from inhalation, smoking and ingesting contaminated food and water [41, 42]. Another source of environmental contamination is landfills, which have been observed to contain levels of cadmium exceeding safety standards in certain cases [43]. Additionally, ingesting this metal from contaminated food has been noted as a typical source of exposure [14, 44].

Exposure to cadmium has been associated with carcinogenesis in multiple tissues including breast, esophagus, stomach, intestines, prostate, lungs and testes [41, 45, 46]. Cadmium also has a proposed role in the development of cancer in the gallbladder. The composition of gallstones, which are recognized as a risk factor for carcinogenesis, were analyzed from patients with this type of cancer [47]. Statistically higher concentrations of cadmium, along with other heavy metals, were observed [47]. Although a causal link involving cadmium was not observed, it does suggest a potential role in malignant growth of the bladder [47]. Cadmium has also demonstrated carcinogenic activity on liver cells in a laboratory setting [44]. Additionally, increased concentrations of cadmium were detected in patients with malignant gliomas, suggesting a potential role of carcinogenesis in the brain [48]. Another organ where cadmium is suggested to exert carcinogenic influence is the pancreas [15, 49]. This metal also has a suspected association with the development of chronic myeloid and lymphoblastic leukemia. It was determined that, when compared to controls, patients with these forms of leukemia displayed significantly elevated concentrations of cadmium and lower levels of magnesium in blood and serum samples [50]. Further work with this metal determined that increased concentration of cadmium in urine was strongly correlated with risk of developing gastrointestinal cancer [51].

Similar to other heavy metals, carcinogenic mechanisms associated with cadmium include generation of ROS, epigenetic alterations, inhibiting DNA repair processes and apoptosis [41, 46, 52, 53]. It has been demonstrated that both chronic and acute cadmium exposure has the ability to induce changes in gene regulation, which generates an increased risk for malignant growth [44]. Key proteins that displayed upregulated expression include DNAJB9, a protein involved in regulating cell destruction, and metallothioneins [44]. Important regulatory proteins also displayed downregulated expression, such as EGR-1, a protein involved in regulating transcription [44]. There are not currently any standard therapeutic measures for the treatment of cadmium poisoning [54]. However, there is ongoing research to develop compounds that reduce the toxic effects of this metal. For example there has been research to develop unique peptoid ligands with selective affinity for cadmium [54]. It has also been determined that flavonoids, compounds present in most plants, have antioxidant properties and can chelate cadmium atoms [55]. Further study is recommended to determine how the structure of flavonoids relates to its action on cadmium [55]. There is also investigation into the use of stem cells as a therapeutic measure for cadmium induced damage. For one study, rat testes were subjected to damaging levels of cadmium [56]. Upon treatment with bone marrow mesenchymal stem cells, it was observed that the rat testes displayed more appropriate levels of proteins related to apoptosis regulation [56]. Additionally, these cells were determined to restore damaged testes tissue, and it was suggested that a possible mechanism is associated with mitochondrial apoptosis [56].

6. Lead

Lead is a toxic heavy metal and exposure constitutes significant risks to health. One common source of environmental pollution has been found in the soil, which can enter the human food cycle through contaminated produce [57–59]. Despite being banned from use in commercially available gasoline in 1995, lead is still added to aviation fuel [59]. This source of environmental pollution has been determined to contribute high emission levels of lead [59]. It was also determined that smokers contained elevated levels of blood lead, representing an additional source of environmental exposure [60]. Certain occupations also play a role in lead exposure, such as mining [57].

Various epidemiological studies have been performed to determine if increased lead exposure is associated with any forms of cancer. Additionally, current research has indicated at this point that lead may not have a causal role in cancer, but it may play a more supportive role [61]. Along with cadmium, lead was detected in significantly higher concentrations in glioma patients, suggesting these two metals combined may produce excessively toxic effects [48]. One study has determined strong correlation between lead exposure and the development of kidney cancer [58]. Another study concluded that patients with higher levels of blood lead had an increased risk of developing renal cell carcinoma [60]. Lead was one of several heavy metals observed in statistically higher concentrations in gallstones [47]. This suggests exposure to this metal represents an increased risk of malignant growth in the gallbladder [47]. In a study performed on lead exposed workers, positive correlation was observed between exposure to this heavy metal and increased risk of carcinogenesis in lung tissue and marginal positive correlation for malignant growth in brain, larynx and bladder tissues [62]. Along with several additional heavy metals, lead was reportedly detected in elevated levels in individuals with exocrine pancreatic cancer, suggesting an unknown mechanism in the development of this cancer [15].

Current literature has not displayed a comprehensive understanding of carcinogenic mechanisms of lead; however, plausible mechanisms have been proposed. Based on the present understanding of lead, it was hypothesized to support the carcinogenic process by disrupting cellular tumor regulation genes, the DNA repair system and inducing DNA damage [63]. In a study performed on mice, there was evidence to support lead's role in generating ROS and altering chromosomal structure and sequence [63]. It was also determined that lead had the potential to disrupt the transcription process by replacing zinc in certain proteins that regulate this system [63]. In an epidemiological study, it was determined that elevated levels of serum calcium were correlated with lower risk of developing renal cell carcinoma, which suggested the need for a clinical trial to determine significance [60]. Chelation therapy is the recommended course of action for individuals with lead poisoning [64]. Common chelators for reducing levels of lead in the body include British, Anti-Lewisite, calcium disodium ethylenediaminetetraacetic acid, D-penicillamine and Meso-2,3-dimercaptosuccinic acid, and use of a specific chelator depends on the situation of the individual [64]. There has also been research into the effectiveness of less toxic therapies. For instance, when garlic was administered in a clinical setting, it was found to reduce blood lead levels in non-severe lead poisoning and alleviate symptoms [64]. The most effective strategy for keeping blood concentration of lead low is prevention of exposure [58]. This includes ensuring that industries that generate significant levels of lead emissions and employees follow safety guidelines for limiting exposure [64]. It has also been suggested that identification of lead contamination sources, followed by removal or avoidance, constitutes the ideal solution to reduce exposure to this heavy metal [64].

7. Mercury

Mercury is another toxic heavy metal with the potential for serious health complications. Although this element can be found in trace amounts in mineral form, most present in the environment is due to human induced pollution from processed mercury [65]. Mercury has a wide range of uses that result in occupational and environmental contamination. Several sources of this heavy metal have been identified as thermometers, fossil fuel emissions, dental fillings, certain batteries and burning medical waste [65, 66]. Mercury compounds have the potential to be vaporized and enter the atmosphere or leech into soil or water systems [65, 67]. Consuming large quantities of seafood has been identified as a primary method for environmental exposure to methyl mercury [65]. Although the pathway through which mercury enters the ecosystem has not been discovered, bioaccumulation of this heavy metal has been observed in shellfish and tuna [65, 68, 69].

Although a causal role has not been established at this time, it has been proposed that mercury exposure may be associated with renal cancer due to this organ being a target for this element [65]. Another study observed that increased mercury exposure has been correlated with liver cancer, and it also has the carcinogenic potential to induce gastric cancer [70]. Mercury was another heavy metal detected in gallstones in statistically higher concentrations from patients with gallbladder cancer [47]. A causal association was not observed with this metal, but a role in carcinogenic development was hypothesized [47].

Comparable to most of the other heavy metals discussed in this study, mercury has the potential to induce malignant growth through several specific mechanisms. These include the ability to generate free radicals as well as disrupt DNA molecular structure and the maintenance system [66]. However, there have been several proposed carcinogenic mechanisms of mercury that are either unique to this metal or not observed in most heavy metals. One mechanism that enhances the carcinogenicity of mercury is its role in reducing the body's concentration of glutathione, a natural antioxidant [71]. This could potentially contribute to increasing susceptibility of essential cellular components to oxidative stress. Oxidative stress on cells has been shown to elevate rates of lipid peroxidation, another mechanism associated with carcinogenesis [65]. It has also been proposed that mercury can affect the microtubules in cells, which, among other processes, can disrupt cellular division [66]. The use of chelators is the common therapeutic strategy for eliminating mercury from the body. It has been determined that the two most effective chelators in a clinical setting are dimercaptosuccinic acid (DMSA) and dimercaptopropane sulfonate (DMPS) [72, 73]. There has also been research to investigate untested chelators for their effectiveness against mercury. For instance, deferasirox and deferiprone were combined and tested on rats [74]. It was observed that this combination was able to successfully chelate mercury and reduced toxic effects of mercury [74]. One unique experimental chelator was thiol-modified nanoporous silica material [75]. Following animal testing, it was observed that this material displayed tremendous potential for eliminating mercury, along with several other heavy metals, with marginal toxicity [75].

8. Nickel

Nickel, a heavy metal present in Earth's core, has garnered research attention due to increased understanding of carcinogenic properties. This metal can produce toxic effects upon exposure in an environmental or occupational setting. Several industries involving potential occupational exposure to nickel include mining, metal alloys and the refinement of nickel [76–78]. Pollution of this heavy metal can enter the environment and bioaccumulate in organisms that enter the human food chain, such as fish [79]. Contaminated soil represents another method of contacting this toxic metal [76]. Emissions from oil refineries have also been established as a significant source of nickel pollution, creating risk for environmental exposure to residents in close proximity [80].

There are a variety of cancers that have been associated with nickel exposure. Epidemiological studies have revealed a significant correlation between exposure and the incidence of carcinogenesis in lung, nasal and sinus tissues [13, 77, 81, 82]. In another study, high levels of serum nickel were determined to be statistically significant in patients with breast cancer, suggesting that exposure has potentially carcinogenic consequences [83]. Exposure to this heavy metal has also been associated with the development of acute myeloid and lymphoblastic leukemia. It was determined that urine contained higher levels of nickel and 8-hydroxy-2′-deoxyguanosine in children with this leukemia [84]. These results suggested a role of nickel in acute leukemia by inducing oxidative damage as a mechanism of action [84]. Research has also revealed the presence of elevated nickel concentrations in individuals with exocrine pancreatic cancer [15]. Although there were other heavy metals present, these findings suggest carcinogenic action from nickel [15]. Another study proposed a link between chronic allergic stimulation from several heavy metals, including nickel, and the development of cutaneous T-cell lymphoma [85]. Furthermore, significant correlation was observed between exposure and mortality rates of liver cancer [13].

Nickel has an extensive range of carcinogenic mechanisms. One such mechanism involves its role in affecting the expression of specific long noncoding RNAs. It has been determined that nickel possesses the ability to induce the downregulation of maternally expressed gene 3 (MEG3) through the methylation of its related promoter [81]. This process was shown to inhibit expression of PHLPP1 and upregulate hypoxia-inducible factor-1α, two proteins recognized for their role in carcinogenesis [81]. It has also been demonstrated that nickel can generate free radicals, which contributes to the carcinogenic process [86]. Exposure to this heavy metal also has the ability to alter the regulation status for the transcription of various mRNAs and microRNAs [78]. The expression of these transcripts has roles in immunity as well as inflammation, which both have proposed roles in the development of malignant growth [78].

The role of nickel in chronic inflammation was investigated in animals and samples of human cells. It was concluded that exposure elevated expression of proteins SQSTM1 and TNF, which have roles in maintaining levels of inflammation, and induced carcinogenesis [82]. Like other heavy metals, nickel has the potential to induce epigenetic changes such as alterations in DNA methylation. For instance, it was observed that nickel ions (Ni2+) had the potential to induce the tri-methylation of histone H3K4 [87]. This process has been correlated with inappropriate transcriptional activation, which suggests another carcinogenic mechanism for nickel [87]. Compared to other heavy metals, the use of chelators involving nickel has been markedly different. Sodium diethyldithiocarbamate has proven to be an effective chelator in response to nickel carbonyl, but a chelator associated with nickel cancer has not been recommended at this point [88]. Despite this fact, there has been research into the use of chelators to remove nickel from the environment. For instance, it was observed that ethylene diamine tetraacetic acid (EDTA) induces the uptake of nickel from contaminated soil in *Arundo donax* L. [89]. This carries tremendous potential for use in areas where nickel is present in dangerous concentrations. It was also determined that CaNa(2) EDTA reverses the damage induced by nickel chloride as well as eliminate the metal from Cirrhinus mrigala [90].

9. Radium

Radium is a radioactive heavy metal that can negatively impact health. This ionizing radiation results from radium decaying into toxic radon gas [91]. Occupational and environmental presence of radium generates opportunities for exposure to ionizing radiation. Coal mining has been noted as one of the most relevant occupations with risk for exposure [92]. Wastewater drained from mines also carries potential for environmental radium contamination [92]. Radium presents further occupational hazards from exposure sources that include soil, building materials and water systems [93]. A study performed in Italy suggested radon gas tends to concentrate in confined spaces of buildings, such as basements or storage areas [91]. Due to radon's ability to bind to cigarette smoke, it was observed that this act increased the accumulation of radon inside buildings [93]. This suggests that smoking increases radium's impact as an environmental contaminant.

Radium is a known carcinogen that is associated with several cancers. Since a primary method of exposure to radon gas has been identified as inhalation, radium has been strongly correlated with the development of lung cancer [91]. Due to the radioactive nature of this metal, chelators are generally not necessary. Nevertheless, it has been determined to have several unique uses. For example, radium has been used as a therapy for patients with ankylosing spondylitis. However, injection of this metal was determined to be associated with increased risk of various forms of leukemia [94]. Injection of mice with radium was determined to cause the generation of osteosarcomas [94]. In another particular case, it was proposed that a patient developed a cutaneous squamous cell carcinoma in response to treatment with radium-223 that extravasated [95]. This study suggested that patients with extravasated radioactive substances require the oversight of a dermatologist [95].

10. Conclusion

Heavy metals exhibit an immense range of toxic effects in humans with regard to carcinogenesis. The research available at this point has illuminated several areas of emphasis for future work. It is clear that a refined understanding of carcinogenic mechanisms is necessary. This could help generate personalized therapeutic or prevention measures for specific heavy metals. Continued consolidation of information is another essential factor moving forward. Effective educational programs are also needed in high-risk areas to raise awareness of the risks associated with exposure to heavy metals.

Author details

Austin Carver and Vincent S. Gallicchio*

*Address all correspondence to: vsgall@clemson.edu

Department of Biological Sciences, College of Science, Clemson University, Clemson, South Carolina, United States of America

References

[1] Mandriota SJ, Tenan M, Ferrari P, Sappino AP. Aluminium chloride promotes tumorigenesis and metastasis in normal murine mammary gland epithelial cells. International Journal of Cancer. 2016;**139**(12):2781-2790. DOI: 10.1002/ijc.30393

[2] Darbre PD. Aluminium and the human breast. Morphologie. 2016;**100**(329):65-74. DOI: 10.1016/j.morpho.2016.02.001

[3] Farasani A, Darbre PD. Effects of aluminium chloride and aluminium chlorohydrate on DNA repair in MCF10A immortalised non-transformed human breast epithelial cells. Journal of Inorganic Biochemistry. 2015;**152**:186-189. DOI: 10.1016/j.jinorgbio.2015.08.003

[4] Roncati L, Gatti AM, Capitani F, Barbolini G, Maiorana A, Palmieri B. Heavy metal bioaccumulation in an atypical primitive neuroectodermal tumor of the abdominal wall. Ultrastructural Pathology. 2015;**39**(4):286-292. DOI: 10.3109/01913123.2015.1013655

[5] Abdel-Gawad M, Elsobky E, Shalaby MM, Abd-Elhameed M, Abdel-Rahim M, Ali-El-Dein B. Quantitative evaluation of heavy metals and trace elements in the urinary bladder: Comparison between cancerous, adjacent non-cancerous and normal cadaveric tissue. Biological Trace Element Research. 2016;**174**(2):280-286. DOI: 10.1007/s12011-016-0764-6

[6] Yokel RA. Aluminum chelation: Chemistry, clinical, and experimental studies and the search for alternatives to desferrioxamine. Journal of Toxicology and Environmental Health. 1994;**41**(2):131-174. DOI: 10.1080/15287399409531834

[7] Ambiado K, Bustos C, Schwarz A, Bórquez R. Membrane technology applied to acid mine drainage from copper mining. Water Science and Technology. 2016;**75**(3):705-715. DOI: 10.2166/wst.2016.556

[8] Martinez VD, Vucic EA, Becker-Santos DD, Gil L, Lam WL. Arsenic exposure and the induction of human cancers. Journal of Toxicology. 2011;**2011**:1-13. DOI: 10.1155/2011/431287

[9] Bjørklund G, Aaseth J, Chirumbolo S, Urbina MA, Uddin R. Effects of arsenic toxicity beyond epigenetic modifications. Environmental Geochemistry and Health. 2017;**39**:1-11 DOI: 10.1007/s10653-017-9967-9

[10] Chakraborti D, Das B, Rahman MM, Nayak B, Pal A, Sengupta MK, Ahamed S, Hossain MA, Chowdhury UK, Biswas BK, Saha KC, Dutta RN. Arsenic in groundwater of the Kolkata Municipal Corporation (KMC), India: Critical review and modes of mitigation. Chemosphere. 2017;**180**:437-447. DOI: 10.1016/j.chemosphere.2017.04.051

[11] Nachman KE, Ginsberg GL, Miller MD, Murray CJ, Nigra AE, Pendergrast CB. Mitigating dietary arsenic exposure: Current status in the United States and recommendations for an improved path forward. Science of the Total Environment. 2017;**581-582**:221-236. DOI: 10.1016/j.scitotenv.2016.12.112

[12] Pershagen G. The carcinogenicity of arsenic. Environmental Health Perspectives. 1981;**40**:93-100. DOI: 10.2307/3429223

[13] Chen K, Liao QL, Ma ZW, Jin Y, Hua M, Bi J, Huang L. Association of soil arsenic and nickel exposure with cancer mortality rates, a town-scale ecological study in Suzhou, China. Environmental Science and Pollution Research. 2014;**22**(7):5395-5404. DOI: 10.1007/s11356-014-3790-y

[14] Satarug S, Vesey DA, Gobe GC. Kidney cadmium toxicity, diabetes and high blood pressure: The perfect storm. The Tohoku Journal of Experimental Medicine. 2017;**241**(1):65-87. DOI: 10.1620/tjem.241.65

[15] Amaral AF, Porta M, Silverman DT, Milne RL, Kogevinas M, Rothman N, Cantor KP, Jackson BP, Pumarega JA, López T, Carrato A, Guarner L, Real FX, Malats N. Pancreatic cancer risk and levels of trace elements. Gut. 2011;**61**(11):1583-1588. DOI: 10.1620/tjem.241.65

[16] Cui J, Xu W, Chen J, Li H, Dai L, Frank JA, Peng S, Wang S, Chen G. M2 polarization of macrophages facilitates arsenic-induced cell transformation of lung epithelial cells. Oncotarget. 2017;**8**(13):21398-21409. DOI: 10.18632/oncotarget.15232

[17] Park YH, Kim D, Dai J, Zhang Z. Human bronchial epithelial BEAS-2B cells, an appropriate in vitro model to study heavy metals induced carcinogenesis. Toxicology and Applied Pharmacology. 2015;**287**(3):240-245. DOI: 10.1016/j.taap.2015.06.008

[18] Hall MN, Niedzwiecki M, Liu X, Harper KN, Alam S, Slavkovich V, Ilievski V, Levy D, Siddique S, Parvez F, Mey JL, van Geen A, Graziano J, Gamble MV. Chronic arsenic exposure and blood glutathione and glutathione disulfide concentrations in

Bangladeshi adults. Environmental Health Perspectives. 2013;**121**(9):1068-1074. DOI: 10.1289/ehp.1205727

[19] Sykora P, Snow ET. Modulation of DNA polymerase beta-dependent base excision repair in cultured human cells after low dose exposure to arsenite. Toxicology and Applied Pharmacology. 2008;**228**(3):385-394. DOI: 10.1016/j.taap.2007.12.019

[20] He J, Wang F, Luo F, Chen X, Jiang W, Huang Z, Lei J, Shan F, Xu X. Effects of long term low- and high-dose sodium arsenite exposure in human transitional cells. American Journal of Translational Research. 2017;**9**(2):416-428

[21] Harper LK, Bayse CA. Modeling the chelation of As(III) in lewisite by dithiols using density functional theory and solvent-assisted proton exchange. Journal of Inorganic Biochemistry. 2015;**153**:60-67. DOI: 10.1016/j.jinorgbio.2015.10.004

[22] Lu PH, Tseng JC, Chen CK, Chen CH. Survival without peripheral neuropathy after massive acute arsenic poisoning: Treated by 2,3-dimercaptopropane-1-sulphonate. Journal of Clinical Pharmacy and Therapeutics. 2017;**42**(4):506-508. DOI: 10.1111/jcpt.12538

[23] Mandal P. Molecular insight of arsenic-induced carcinogenesis and its prevention. Naunyn-Schmiedeberg's Archives of Pharmacology. 2017;**390**(5):443-455. DOI: 10.1007/s00210-017-1351-x

[24] Stanton BA, Caldwell K, Congdon CB, Disney J, Donahue M, Ferguson E, Flemings E, Golden M, Guerinot ML, Highman J, James K, Kim C, Lantz RC, Marvinney RG, Mayer G, Miller D, Navas-Acien A, Nordstrom DK, Postema S, Rardin L, Rosen B, Sengupta A, Shaw J, Stanton E, Susca P. MDI biological laboratory arsenic summit: Approaches to limiting human exposure to arsenic. Current Environmental Health Reports. 2015;**2**(3):329-337. DOI: 10.1007/s40572-015-0057-9

[25] Spanu A, Daga L, Orlandoni AM, Sanna G. The role of irrigation techniques in arsenic bioaccumulation in rice (*Oryza sativa* L.). Environmental Science & Technology. 2012;**46**(15):8333-8340. DOI: 10.1021/es300636d

[26] Nogaj E, Kwapulinski J, Misiołek M, Golusiński W, Kowol J, Wiechuła D. Beryllium concentration in pharyngeal tonsils in children. Annals of Agricultural and Environmental Medicine. 2014;**21**(2):267-271. DOI: 10.5604/1232-1966.1108589

[27] Shay E, De Gandiaga E, Madl AK. Considerations for the development of healthbased surface dust cleanup criteria for beryllium. Critical Reviews in Toxicology. 2013;**43**(3):220-243. DOI: 10.3109/10408444.2013.767308

[28] Boffetta P, Fryzek JP, Mandel JS. Occupational exposure to beryllium and cancer risk: A review of the epidemiologic evidence. Critical Reviews in Toxicology. 2012;**42**(2):107-118. DOI: 10.3109/10408444.2011.631898

[29] Hollins DM, McKinley MA, Williams C, Wiman A, Fillos D, Chapman PS, Madl AK. Beryllium and lung cancer: A weight of evidence evaluation of the toxicological and epidemiological literature. Critical Reviews in Toxicology. 2009;**39**(1):1-32. DOI: 10.1080/10408440902837967

[30] Beryllium and Beryllium Compounds. International Agency for Research on Cancer. 2012;**100C**:95-120

[31] Stark M, Lerman Y, Kapel A, Pardo A, Schwarz Y, Newman L, Maier L, Fireman E. Biological exposure metrics of beryllium-exposed dental technicians. Archives of Environmental & Occupational Health. 2013;**69**(2):89-99. DOI: 10.1080/19338244.2012.744736

[32] Benderli Cihan Y, Sözen S, Oztürk Yıldırım S. Trace elements and heavy metals in hair of stage III breast cancer patients. Biological Trace Element Research. 2011;**144**(1-3):360-379. DOI: 10.1007/s12011-011-9104-z

[33] Sandhu R, Lal H, Kundu ZS, Kharb S. Serum fluoride and sialic acid levels in osteosarcoma. Biological Trace Element Research. 2009;**144**(1-3):1-5. DOI: 10.1007/s12011-009-8382-1

[34] Radauceanu A, Grzebyk M, Edmé JL, Chérot-Kornobis N, Rousset D, Dziurla M, De Broucker V, Hédelin G, Sobaszek A, Hulo S. Effects of occupational exposure to poorly soluble forms of beryllium on biomarkers of pulmonary response in exhaled breath of workers in machining industries. Toxicology Letters. 2016;**263**:26-33. DOI: 10.1016/j.toxlet.2016.10.013

[35] Shukla S, Sharma P, Johri S, Mathur R. Influence of chelating agents on the toxicity and distribution of beryllium in rats. Journal of Applied Toxicology. 1998;**18**(5):331-335. DOI: 10.1002/(SICI)1099-1263(1998090)18:5<331::AID-JAT517>3.0.CO;2-0

[36] Johri S, Shukla S, Sharma P. Role of chelating agents and antioxidants in beryllium induced toxicity. Indian Journal of Experimental Biology. 2002;**40**(5):575-582

[37] Sharma P, Johri S, Shukla S. Beryllium-induced toxicity and its prevention by treatment with chelating agents. Journal of Applied Toxicology. 2000;**20**(4):313-318. DOI: 10.1002/1099-1263(200007/08)20:4<313::AID-JAT660>3.0.CO;2-J

[38] Crinnion WJ, Tran JQ. Case report: Heavy metal burden presenting as Bartter syndrome. Alternative Medicine Review. 2010;**15**(4):303-310

[39] Mayer AS, Brazile WJ, Erb SA, Barker EA, Miller CM, Mroz MM, Maier LA, Van Dyke MV. Developing effective health and safety training materials for workers in beryllium-using industries. Journal of Occupational and Environmental Medicine. 2013;**55**(7):746-751. DOI: 10.1097/JOM.0b013e3182972f1b

[40] Thomas CA, Deubner DC, Stanton ML, Kreiss K, Schuler CR. Long-term efficacy of a program to prevent beryllium disease. American Journal of Industrial Medicine. 2013;**56**(7):733-741. DOI: 10.1002/ajim.22175

[41] Bertin G, Averbeck D. Cadmium: Cellular effects, modifications of biomolecules, modulation of DNA repair and genotoxic consequences (a review). Biochimie. 2006;**88**(11):1549-1559. DOI: 10.1016/j.biochi.2006.10.001

[42] Chunhabundit R. Cadmium exposure and potential health risk from foods in contaminated area, Thailand. Toxicological Research. 2016;**32**(1):65-72. DOI: 10.5487/TR.2016.32.1.065

[43] Alimba CG, Gandhi D, Sivanesan S, Bhanarkar MD, Naoghare PK, Bakare AA, Krishnamurthi K. Chemical characterization of simulated landfill soil leachates from Nigeria and India and their cytotoxicity and DNA damage inductions on three human cell lines. Chemosphere. 2016;**164**:469-479. DOI: 10.1016/j.chemosphere.2016.08.093

[44] Cartularo L, Laulicht F, Sun H, Kluz T, Freedman JH, Costa M. Gene expression and pathway analysis of human hepatocellular carcinoma cells treated with cadmium. Toxicology and Applied Pharmacology. 2015;**288**(3):399-408. DOI: 10.1016/j.taap.2015.08.011

[45] Larsson SC, Orsini N, Wolk A. Urinary cadmium concentration and risk of breast cancer: A systematic review and dose-response meta-analysis. American Journal of Epidemiology. 2015;**182**(5):375-380. DOI: 10.1093/aje/kwv085

[46] Bishak YK, Payahoo L, Osatdrahimi A, Nourazarian A. Mechanisms of cadmium carcinogenicity in the gastrointestinal tract. Asian Pacific Journal of Cancer Prevention. 2015;**16**(1):9-21. DOI: 10.7314/APJCP.2015.16.1.9

[47] Mondal B, Maulik D, Mandal M, Sarkar GN, Sengupta S, Ghosh D. Analysis of carcinogenic heavy metals in gallstones and its role in gallbladder carcinogenesis. Journal of Gastrointestinal Cancer. 2016;1-8. DOI: 10.1007/s12029-016-9898-1

[48] Arslan M, Demir H, Arslan H, Gokalp AS, Demir C. Trace elements, heavy metals and other biochemical parameters in malignant glioma patients. Asian Pacific Journal of Cancer Prevention. 2011;**12**(2):447-451

[49] García-Esquinas E, Pollan M, Tellez-Plaza M, Francesconi KA, Goessler W, Guallar E, Umans JG, Yeh J, Best LG, Navas-Acien A. Cadmium exposure and cancer mortality in a prospective cohort: The strong heart study. Environmental Health Perspectives. 2014;**122**(4):363-370. DOI: 10.1289/ehp.1306587

[50] Khan N, Afridi HI, Kazi TG, Arain MB, Bilal M, Akhtar A, Khan M. Correlation of cadmium and magnesium in the blood and serum samples of smokers and nonsmokers chronic leukemia patients. Biological Trace Element Research. 2016;**176**(1):81-88. DOI: 10.1007/s12011-016-0816-y

[51] Ostadrahimi A, Payahoo L, Somi MH, Khajebishak Y. The association between urinary cadmium levels and dietary habits with risk of gastrointestinal cancer in Tabriz, Northwest of Iran. Biological Trace Element Research. 2016;**175**(1):72-78. DOI: 10.1007/s12011-016-0764-6

[52] Xiao CL, Liu Y, Tu W, Xia YJ, Tian KM, Zhou X. Research progress of the mechanisms underlying cadmium-induced carcinogenesis. Zhonghua Yu Fang Yi Xue Za Zhi. 2016;**50**(4):380-384. DOI: 10.3760/cma.j.issn.0253-9624.2016.04.021

[53] Inglot P, Lewinska A, Potocki L, Oklejewicz B, Tabecka-Lonczynska A, Koziorowski M, Bugno-Poniewierska M, Bartosz G, Wnuk M. Cadmium-induced changes in genomic DNA-methylation status increase aneuploidy events in a pig Robertsonian translocation model. Mutation Research/Genetic Toxicology and Environmental Mutagenesis. 2012;**747**(2):182-189. DOI: 10.1016/j.mrgentox.2012.05.007

[54] Knight AS, Zhou EY, Francis MB. Development of peptoid-based ligands for the removal of cadmium from biological media. Chemical Science. 2015;**6**(7):4042-4048. DOI: 10.1039/C5SC00676G

[55] Li X, Jiang X, Sun J, Zhu C, Li X, Tian L, Liu L, Bai W. Cytoprotective effects of dietary flavonoids against cadmium-induced toxicity. Annals of the New York Academy of Sciences. 2017;**1398**:5-19. DOI: 10.1111/nyas.13344

[56] Wang YJ, Yan J, Zou XL, Guo KJ, Zhao Y, Meng CY, Yin F, Guo L. Bone marrow mesenchymal stem cells repair cadmium-induced rat testis injury by inhibiting mitochondrial apoptosis. Chemico-Biological Interactions. 2017;**271**:39-47. DOI: 10.1016/j.cbi.2017.04.024

[57] Orisakwe OE, Dagur EA, Mbagwu HO, Udowelle NA. Lead levels in vegetables from artisanal mining sites of Dilimi River, Bukuru and Barkin Ladi North Central Nigeria: Cancer and non-cancer risk assessment. Asian Pacific Journal of Cancer Prevention. 2017;**18**(3):621-627. DOI: 10.22034/APJCP.2017.18.3.621

[58] Rashidi M, Alavipanah S. Relation between kidney cancer and soil leads in Isfahan Province, Iran between 2007 and 2009. Journal of Cancer Research and Therapeutics. 2016;**12**(2):716-720. DOI: 10.4103/0973-1482.154936

[59] McCumber A, Strevett KA. A geospatial analysis of soil lead concentrations around regional Oklahoma Airports. Chemosphere. 2017;**167**:62-70. DOI: 10.1016/j.chemosphere.2016.09.127

[60] Southard EB, Roff A, Fortugno T, Richie JP, Kaag M, Chinchilli VM, Virtamo J, Albanes D, Weinstein S, Wilson RT. Lead, calcium uptake, and related genetic variants in association with renal cell carcinoma risk in a cohort of male Finnish smokers. Cancer Epidemiology Biomarkers & Prevention. 2011;**21**(1):191-201. DOI: 10.1158/1055-9965.EPI-11-0670

[61] Silbergeld EK. Facilitative mechanisms of lead as a carcinogen. Mutation Research/Fundamental and Molecular Mechanisms of Mutagenesis. 2003;**533**(1-2):121-133. DOI: 10.1016/j.mrfmmm.2003.07.010

[62] Steenland K, Barry V, Anttila A, Sallmén M, Mcelvenny D, Todd AC, Straif K. A cohort mortality study of lead-exposed workers in the USA, Finland and the UK. Occupational and Environmental Medicine. 2017;May 2017. DOI: 10.1136/oemed-2017-104311

[63] Silbergeld EK, Waalkes M, Rice JM. Lead as a carcinogen: Experimental evidence and mechanisms of action. American Journal of Industrial Medicine. 2000;**38**(3):316-323. DOI: 10.1002/1097-0274(200009)38:3<316::AID-AJIM11>3.0.CO;2-P

[64] Kianoush S, Sadegehi M, Balali-Mood M. Recent advances in the clinical management of lead poisoning. Acta Medica Iranica. 2015;**53**(6):327-336

[65] Rice KM, Walker EM, Wu M, Gillette C, Blough ER. Environmental mercury and its toxic effects. Journal of Preventive Medicine & Public Health. 2014;**47**(2):74-83. DOI: 10.3961/jpmph.2014.47.2.74

[66] Crespo-López ME, Macêdo GL, Pereira SI, Arrifano GP, Picanço-Diniz DL, do Nascimento JL, Herculano AM. Mercury and human genotoxicity: Critical considerations and possible molecular mechanisms. Pharmacological Research. 2009;**60**(4):212-220. DOI: 10.1016/j.phrs.2009.02.011

[67] Branco V, Caito S, Farina M, Rocha J, Aschner M, Carvalho C. Biomarkers of mercury toxicity: Past, present, and future trends. Journal of Toxicology and Environmental Health, Part B. 2017;**20**(3):119-154. DOI: 10.1080/10937404.2017.1289834

[68] Junqué E, Garí M, Arce A, Torrent M, Sunyer J, Grimalt JO. Integrated assessment of infant exposure to persistent organic pollutants and mercury via dietary intake in a central western Mediterranean site (Menorca Island). Environmental Research. 2017;**156**:714-724. DOI: 10.1016/j.envres.2017.04.030

[69] Alcala-Orozco M, Morillo-Garcia Y, Caballero-Gallardo K, Olivero-Verbel J. Mercury in canned tuna marketed in Cartagena, Colombia and estimation of human exposure. Food Additives & Contaminants: Part B. 2017;**10**:1-7. DOI: 10.1080/19393210.2017.1323803

[70] Yuan W, Yang N, Li X. Advances in understanding how heavy metal pollution triggers gastric cancer. BioMed Research International. 2016;**2016**:1-10. DOI: 10.1155/2016/7825432

[71] Valko M, Morris H, Cronin MT. Metals, toxicity and oxidative stress. Current Medicinal Chemistry. 2005;**12**(10):1161-1208. DOI: 10.2174/0929867053764635

[72] Kosnett MJ. The role of chelation in the treatment of arsenic and mercury poisoning. Journal of Medical Toxicology. 2013;**9**(4):347-354.DOI: 10.1007/s13181-013-0344-5

[73] Sears, ME. Chelation: Harnessing and enhancing heavy metal detoxification—A review. The Scientific World Journal. 2013;**2013**:1-13. DOI: 10.1155/2013/219840

[74] Iranmanesh M, Fatemi SJ, Golbafan MR, Balooch FD. Treatment of mercury vapor toxicity by combining deferasirox and deferiprone in rats. BioMetals. 2013;**26**(5):783-788. DOI: 10.1007/s10534-013-9656-9

[75] Sangvanich T, Morry J, Fox C, Ngamcherdtrakul W, Goodyear S, Castro D, Fryxell GE, Addleman RS, Summers AO, Yantasee W. Novel oral detoxification of mercury, cadmium, and lead with thiol-modified nanoporous silica. ACS Applied Materials & Interfaces. 2014;**6**(8):5483-5493. DOI: 10.1021/am5007707

[76] Ngole-Jeme VM, Fantke P. Ecological and human health risks associated with abandoned gold mine tailings contaminated soil. Plos One. 2017;**12**(2). DOI: 10.1371/journal.pone.0172517

[77] Pavela M, Uitti J, Pukkala E. Cancer incidence among copper smelting and nickel refining workers in Finland. American Journal of Industrial Medicine. 2016;**60**(1):87-95. DOI: 10.1002/ajim.22662

[78] Gölz L, Buerfent BC, Hofmann A, Rühl H, Fricker N, Stamminger W, Oldenburg J, Deschner J, Hoerauf A, Nöthen MM, Schumacher J, Hübner MP, Jäger A. Genome-wide transcriptome induced by nickel in human monocytes. Acta Biomaterialia. 2016;**43**:369-382. DOI: 10.1016/j.actbio.2016.07.047

[79] Plavan G, Jitar O, Teodosiu C, Nicoara M, Micu D, Strungaru SA. Toxic metals in tissues of fishes from the Black Sea and associated human health risk exposure. Environmental Science and Pollution Research. 2017;**24**(8):7776-7787. DOI: 10.1007/s11356-017-8442-6

[80] Harari R, Harari F, Forastiere F. Environmental nickel exposure from oil refinery emissions: A case study in Ecuador. Annali dell'Istituto Superiore di Sanità. 2016;**52**(4):495-499. DOI: 10.4415/ANN_16_04_06

[81] Zhou C, Huang C, Wang J, Huang H, Li J, Xie Q, Liu Y, Zhu J, Li Y, Zhang D, Zhu Q. LncRNA MEG3 downregulation mediated by DNMT3b contributes to nickel malignant transformation of human bronchial epithelial cells via modulating PHLPP1 transcription and HIF-1α translation. Oncogene. 2017;**36**:3878-3889. DOI: 10.1038/onc.2017.14

[82] Huang H, Zhu J, Li Y, Zhang L, Gu J, Xie Q, Jin H, Che X, Li J, Huang C, Chen LC, Lyu J, Gao J, Huang C. Upregulation of SQSTM1/p62 contributes to nickel-induced malignant transformation of human bronchial epithelial cells. Autophagy. 2016;**12**(10):1687-1703. DOI: 10.1080/15548627.2016.1196313

[83] Yu M, Zhang J. Serum and hair nickel levels and breast cancer: Systematic review and meta-analysis. Biological Trace Element Research. 2017:**175**(2):1-7. DOI: 10.1007/s12011-017-0949-7

[84] Yang Y, Jin X, Yan C, Tian Y, Tang J, Shen X. Urinary level of nickel and acute leukaemia in Chinese children. Toxicology and Industrial Health. 2008;**24**(9):603-610. DOI: 10.1177/0748233708100091

[85] Tilakaratne D, Sidhu S. Heavy metal (monoclonal) bands: A link between cutaneous T-cell lymphoma and contact allergy to potassium dichromate, nickel and cobalt? Australasian Journal of Dermatology. 2014;**56**(1):59-63. DOI: 10.1111/ajd.12182

[86] Zambelli B, Uversky VN, Ciurli S. Nickel impact on human health: An intrinsic disorder perspective. Biochimica Et Biophysica Acta (BBA) – Proteins and Proteomics. 2016;**1864**(12):1714-1731. DOI: 10.1016/j.bbapap.2016.09.008

[87] Ma L, Bai Y, Pu H, Gou F, Dai M, Wang H, He J, Zheng T, Cheng N. Histone methylation in nickel-smelting industrial workers. Plos One. 2015;**10**(10). DOI: 10.1371/journal.pone.0140339

[88] Sunderman FW. Chelation therapy in nickel poisoning. Annals of Clinical and Laboratory Science. 1981;**11**(1):1-8

[89] Atma W, Larouci M, Meddah B, Benabdeli K, Sonnet P. Evaluation of the phytoremediation potential of *Arundo donax* L. for nickel-contaminated soil. International Journal of Phytoremediation. 2017;**19**(4):377-386. DOI: 10.1080/15226514.2016.1225291

[90] Gopal R, Narmada S, Vijayakumar R, Jaleel CA. Chelating efficacy of CaNa2 EDTA on nickel-induced toxicity in Cirrhinus mrigala (Ham.) through its effects on glutathione peroxidase, reduced glutathione and lipid peroxidation. Comptes Rendus Biologies. 2009;**332**(8):685-696. DOI: 10.1016/j.crvi.2009.03.004

[91] Di Loreto G, Sacco A, Felicioli G. Radon in workplaces, a review. Giornale Italiano Di Medicina Del Lavoro Ed Ergonomia. 2010;**32**(4):251-254

[92] Chałupnik S, Wysocka M, Janson E, Chmielewska I, Wiesner M. Long term changes in the concentration of radium in sischarge waters of coal mines and Upper Silesian rivers. Journal of Environmental Radioactivity. 2017;**171**:117-123. DOI: 10.1016/j.jenvrad.2017.02.007

[93] Abdel Ghany HA. Enhancement of radon exposure in smoking areas. Environmental Geochemistry and Health. 2007;**29**(3):249-255. DOI: 10.1007/s10653-007-9082-4

[94] Wick RR, Nekolla EA, Gaubitz M, Schulte TL. Increased risk of myeloid leukaemia in patients with ankylosing spondylitis following treatment with radium-224. Rheumatology. 2008;**47**(6):855-859. DOI: 10.1093/rheumatology/ken060

[95] Benejegerdes KE, Brown SC, Housewright CD. Focal cutaneous squamous cell carcinoma following radium-223 extravasation. Proceedings (Baylor University Medical Center). 2017;**30**(1):78-79

Chapter 2

Cancer, Carcinogens and Screening in the Kidney

Michael Higgins, Ismael Obaidi and Tara McMorrow

Additional information is available at the end of the chapter

http://dx.doi.org/10.5772/intechopen.72722

Abstract

This chapter examines a number of different aspects of renal cancer. Firstly, an introduction into the numerous forms of renal cancers is provided, focusing on renal cell carcinomas their causes and the different treatment options currently available. This chapter also takes a look at renal cancer from a toxicological point of view. Due to the crucial role of the kidneys in blood filtration, this allows them to become susceptible to the exposure and accumulation of potentially carcinogenic chemicals. For this reason, renal carcinogens are looked at in detail focusing on the varying mechanisms of genotoxic renal carcinogens such as aristolochic acid and potassium bromate, and their non-genotoxic renal carcinogens counterparts including ochratoxin A and chlorothalonil. This chapter also examines the different methods currently used to detect a compound's carcinogenic potential, including the *in vitro* Ames test and animal based carcinogenicity screening methods.

Keywords: cancer, renal cancer, renal carcinogens, carcinogen screening, genotoxic/non-genotoxic carcinogens

1. Renal cancer

In 2016 alone there was a reported 62,700 cases of cancer involving the kidney and the renal pelvis worldwide [1]. Renal cell carcinoma (RCC) is the most common form of kidney cancer and makes up approximately 90–95% of all kidney cancers [2]. The incidence of RCC has been found to be higher in developed countries and is also more common amongst men, the exact reasons for this are currently unknown [3]. Five year survival rates for stage I RCC is 80–90%, for stage II it is 80%, for stage III it is approximately 60% and stage IV survival is estimated at just 10%. RCCs can be categorised into a number of subgroups; clear cell RCC (ccRCC), papillary RCC and chromophobe RCC [4].

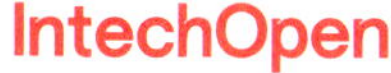

Clear cell RCC (ccRCC) aptly named due to its clear cytoplasm. This clear cytoplasm is caused by its high glycogen and lipid content in the cytosol. ccRCC is the most common form of RCC, making up 70% of all kidney cancer cases [5]. ccRCC are thought to arise from proximal tubular epithelial cells and have a worse prognosis than papillary or chromophobe carcinoma [6, 7]. Approximately 95% of ccRCC are sporadic with the remaining 5% having a familial link [7]. Von Hippel–Lindau (VHL) disease is a hereditary condition that is heavily implicated in the development of familial ccRCC [8]. Mutations in the VHL are implicated in virtually all cases of familial ccRCC and approximately 57% of sporadic ccRCC [9]. Mutations in VHL also lead to the activation of hypoxia-inducible factor-1α (HIF1A) and hypoxia inducible factor-2α (HIF2A). Activation of these HIF related pathways leads to the activation of genes involved in angiogenesis and vascular endothelial growth [6]. The second most commonly mutated gene in ccRCC is polybromo 1 (PBRM1). Mutations in this gene are found in 45% of all ccRCC, its exact role in the development of tumour growth is not well understood, however it is thought that PBRM1s role is in controlling cell proliferation [10]. Components of the PI3K/AKT pathway are also believed to be implicated in ccRCC. In a study of a ccRCC database of 20 PI3K/AKT pathway panel components were assessed, 27% of the components were found to have genetic alterations related to PI3K/AKT pathway [11].

2. Other renal carcinomas

Similar to ccRCC papillary renal carcinomas are thought to arise from the epithelial cells in the proximal tubule [6]. Two hereditary conditions are linked with the development of papillary renal carcinomas, these conditions involve mutations in the MET proto-oncogene and fumarate hydrate genes, respectively [4]. However, this form of renal carcinomas is not well understood.

Chromophobe RCC (chRCC) makes up about 5% of all renal cancers [7]. chRCC is usually found in stage I or II and the tumour usually presents itself as a highly lobulated large mass, with a median tumour size of 6 cm [12]. The exact genetic alterations in chRCC are not well understood, however loss of entire chromosome 2, 10, 13, 17 and 21 occurs in almost all cases of chRCC. It is the least aggressive of all RCCs and for this reason has a low malignancy potential with a 10 year survival rate estimated at 80–90% [13]. Tumour development can also occur in the collecting duct of the kidney. This is a rare form of renal cancer that usually presents itself at an advanced stage and is believed to arise from the epithelial cells in the collecting duct [14].

3. Treatment

Fifty percent of all renal cancers are diagnosed when an ultrasound is carried out for symptoms including abdominal pain, hypertension, weight loss and elevated CRP, due to this difficulty in diagnosing renal cancer about 25% of patients present with cancer that has metastasized [15]. Surgery is commonly used in the treatment of renal cancer, depending on the severity of the disease the nephrectomy can be partial or radical. Radical nephrectomy involves the removal of the entire kidney, the adrenal gland and possibly the regionally located lymph nodes [16]. Although it is seen as an effective treatment of renal cancer, its use is associated with development of chronic kidney disease (CKD) and other cardiovascular related diseases [17]. Partial nephrectomy (also called nephron-sparing surgery) is also used, however this technique is underused due to the technical difficulties involved in removing only a part of the kidney where the tumour is localised. Partial nephrectomy has a 5 year survival rate of 87–90% [2]. Renal cell carcinomas are highly resistant to chemotherapeutic agents, for this reason the currently available drugs involve targeted therapies, including cytokines, mTOR inhibitors and targeting the vascular endothelial growth factor (VEGF) pathway [4]. A number of different cytokine related therapies are available such as interleukin 2 (IL-2) and interferon alpha (IFN-alpha), although these options have anti-cancer ability they are found not to be effective in cases where the tumour has metastasized [18]. The development of RCC is closely linked to a number of different components involved in angiogenesis, for this reason anti-angiogenic therapies have been developed targeting in particular the VEGF pathway, these include bevacizumab, sorafenib and sunitinib. These treatments have replaced interleukin related immunotherapies as a first line treatment following the partial or radical nephrectomy [19]. The mTOR pathway is involved in cell survival and its dysregulation has been shown to be heavily implicated in a number of forms of cancer [20]. Temsirolimus and everolimus, both mTOR inhibitors have been approved by the FDA for treatment of RCC, temsirolimus is considered the first line of treatment for metastatic RCC where the prognosis is poor, everolimus is used where the disease has progressed during treatment with VEGF targeted treatment [21].

4. Carcinogens

In the international agency for research on cancer (IARC) review of human carcinogens, they describe 'the term carcinogenic risk…is taken to mean that an agent is capable of causing cancer' [22]. Carcinogens are capable of inducing the process of carcinogenesis by variety of different mechanisms, these include by genotoxic (directly interacting with DNA) and non-genotoxic (indirectly lead to DNA instability) mechanisms. Carcinogenic factors have been grouped into these different categories; primary and secondary determining factor and favouring factors. Primary determining factors can be defined as a compound or chemical which is capable of inducing cancer by acting on a molecular level. Secondary determining factors are caused by hereditary factors where there is a genetic mutation with a familial link that ultimately results in cancer formation. Lastly, favouring factors are ones that may increase the possibility of tumorigenesis, these include diet, gender, age and possibly geographical location [23]. As well as carcinogens, there are also compounds called co-carcinogens that do not cause cancer by themselves but may increase the carcinogenic ability of other carcinogens [24].

5. Genotoxic vs. non-genotoxic carcinogens

Carcinogens can be classified by their mechanism of carcinogenicity. These categories include genotoxic and non-genotoxic carcinogens (**Figure 1**). In general, genotoxic carcinogens function

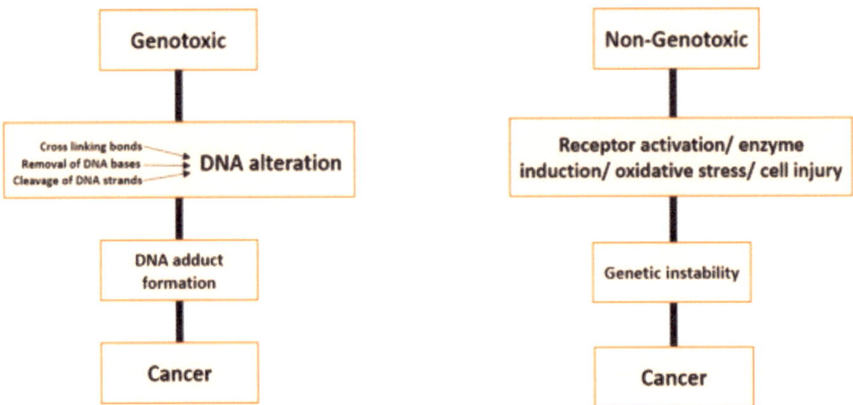

Figure 1. Mechanisms of genotoxicity and non-genotoxicity carcinogenicity. Carcinogens can be categorised as either genotoxic or non-genotoxic carcinogens. Genotoxic carcinogens induce the carcinogenesis process by directly interfering with DNA leading to genetic instability, if DNA replication occurs prior to the repair of the damage. Non-genotoxic carcinogens on the other hand indirectly interfere with DNA, this can occur by a number of mechanisms including ROS production.

by directly interfering with the patients DNA, this causes the formation of covalent bonds and eventually leads to the development of DNA adducts, while non-genotoxic carcinogens do not directly interact with DNA but act in a carcinogenic fashion through other mechanisms. Genotoxic carcinogens are believed to induce DNA damage by the formation of a cross-linking bond between two helices, the removal of DNA bases and the cleavage of DNA strands, all contributing to the alteration of DNA [25]. In general, this DNA damage would be repaired, however if DNA replication occurs before the damage is fixed the mutation may result in cancer development. As all cancers have alterations in DNA expression, non-genotoxic carcinogens are capable of inducing this genetic instability by an indirect manipulation of the natural regulation of DNA expression. In general non-genotoxic carcinogens appear to be more specific than genotoxic carcinogens in their carcinogenic ability, where they are often only capable of inducing cancer in one species, in one organ and sometimes in one sex [26]. Although the mechanisms of non-genotoxic carcinogenicity are less well understood than their genotoxic counterparts, attempts have been made to classify the main mechanisms of non-genotoxic carcinogenicity, these have included receptor activation, CYP450 induction, stimulation of oxidative stress, chronic cell injury, immunosuppression and interference with intercellular communication [26, 27].

6. Genotoxic carcinogens

Examples of genotoxic renal carcinogens are potassium bromate, 2-nitroflourene, benzo-A-pyrene, aristolochic acid and streptozotocin (**Figure 2**). Potassium bromate is a white crystal powder that is listed by the IARC as a group 2B carcinogen. Before its toxicity was established potassium bromate was widely utilised in the food industry, typically used to strengthen

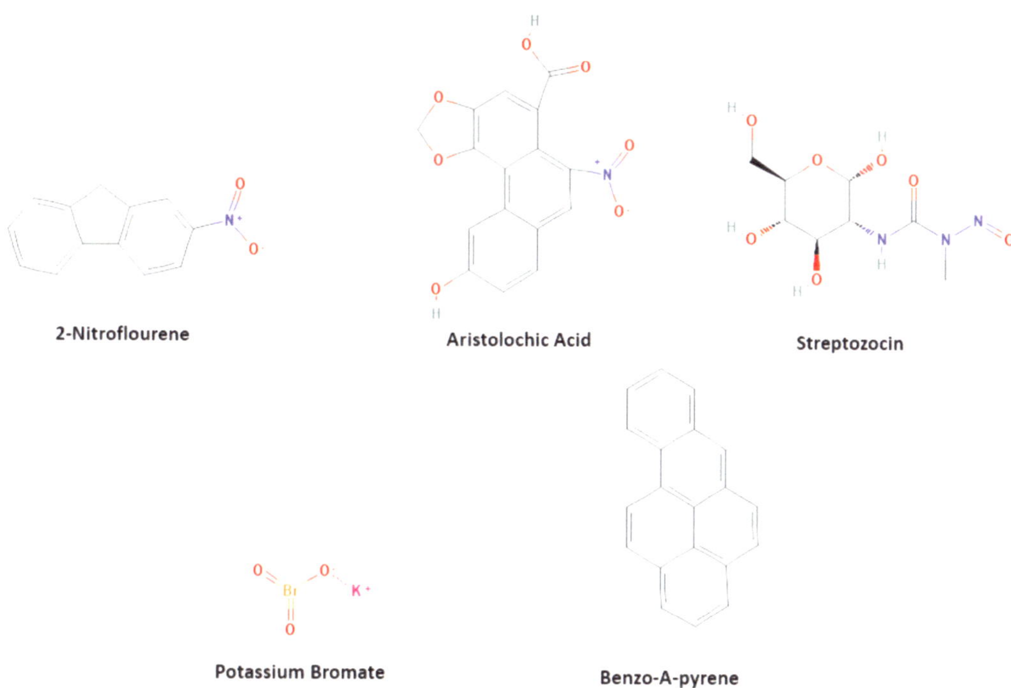

Figure 2. Chemical structure of a number genotoxic renal carcinogens (All chemical structures are adapted from https://www.ncbi.nlm.nih.gov/pccompound).

dough. Potassium bromate is a highly toxic compound that can cause oxidative DNA damage by inducing the formation of 8-hydroxyguanine (oh8Gua) [28]. 2-nitroflourene is found in the emissions from diesel fumes and kerosene heaters. This by-product of combustion is listed as a group 2B carcinogen. It has been shown to be capable of causing DNA adduct formation in rats, thus proving its genotoxicity [29]. Benzo-A-pyrene is another genotoxic carcinogen, listed as a group 1 human carcinogen. It causes a missense mutation in the tumour suppressor p53 [30]. Aristolochic acids are an extract from a plant commonly found in Asia. Plants containing aristolochic acids are classified as group 1 human carcinogens. Aristolochic acids are capable of producing DNA adducts found in tumour tissue of patients with urinary tract cancer in an area of Taiwan where the use of herbal medicine containing aristolochic acids is the most prevalent [31]. Lastly, streptozotocin is a 2B carcinogen with possible carcinogenic ability in humans and has been shown to cause tumour formation in rat kidneys and neoplastic transformation in human primary renal cells [32, 33].

7. Non-genotoxic carcinogens

Non-genotoxic renal carcinogens include ochratoxin A (OTA), monuron, bromodichloromethane and chlorothalonil (**Figure 3**). Ochratoxin A (OTA) is classified by the IARC as a group 2B carcinogen with possible human carcinogenic ability. OTA is a naturally occurring

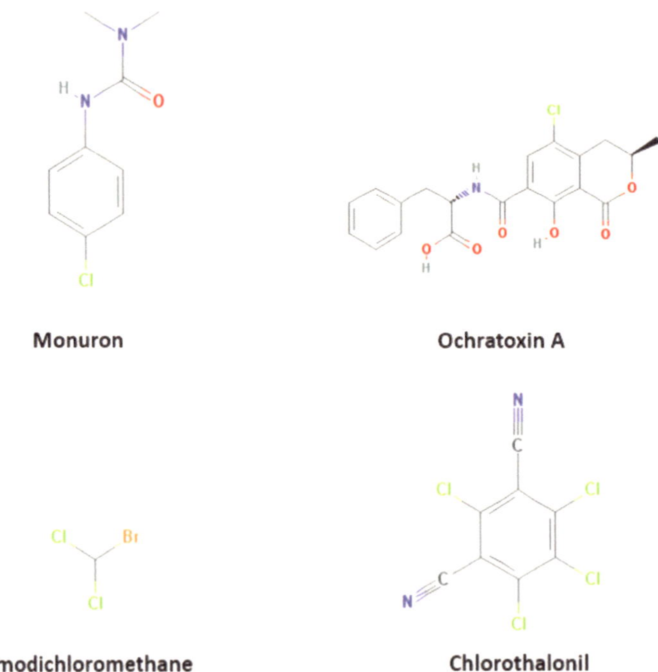

Figure 3. Chemical structure of a number of non-genotoxic renal carcinogens (All chemical structures are adapted from https://www.ncbi.nlm.nih.gov/pccompound).

mycotoxin, OTA causes contamination of food and drink products [34, 35]. OTA exposure is associated with Balkan endemic nephropathy that causes tumour formation in the urinary tract and the kidney [36]. Much work has been carried out to establish whether OTA is a genotoxic or non-genotoxic carcinogen. The formation of DNA adducts following OTA treatment would point to a possible genotoxic mechanism [37]. However, a review by Mally et al. refuted these findings where they claimed that OTA induced DNA adduct formation was not an important mechanism in OTAs overall carcinogenicity [38]. A study by Mantle et al. discussed that the reclassification of a carcinogen from a non-genotoxic to genotoxic has far reaching ramifications in terms of legislation, particularly with a contaminant found in the food and drinks industry, as a non-genotoxic carcinogen is said to have a 10-fold reduced risk to humans compared to genotoxic carcinogens [39]. This being said OTA's ability to induce the formation of reactive oxygen species is the strongest piece of evidence to suggest its non-genotoxicity [40].

Monuron is a phenylurea herbicide and a known renal carcinogen in rats as it has been shown to cause adenomas of the kidney and carcinomas of the liver [41]. In a study by Block et al. they showed that monuron induced an upregulation of genes involved in cell cycle and cell proliferation in the renal cortex [42]. Due to its unclear mechanism of carcinogenicity a number of studies have classified it as a non-genotoxic renal carcinogen [43]. Bromodichloromethane is a trihalomethane and according to the IARC is a proven carcinogen in rats and a suspected human carcinogen (Group 2B). It is also thought to cause some chromosomal aberrations

[44]. Chlorothalonil is a fungicide used in fungal control in a number of different crops. It is classified as a group 2B carcinogen to humans. A report by the *Environmental Protection Agency* in the United States declared that although an exact mechanism of carcinogenicity for chlorothalonil was unestablished it was agreed that the probable mechanism of carcinogenicity was through a non-genotoxic route as it behaved very similarly to other well established non-genotoxic carcinogens [45].

8. Bioactivation of carcinogens

In general cytochrome p450 monooxygenases play the role of detoxifying certain chemicals in the body, the opposite can also occur where these enzymes can bioactivate a particular compound where oxidation causes the conversion into a toxic by-product [46]. 2-acetylaminofluorene, a carcinogen capable of inducing tumour formation in the liver and kidney, is converted by a CYP450 mediated N-hydroxylation to produce a hydroxylamine which undergoes further transformation to become the deadly activated carcinogenic form [47]. Another example of CYP450 induced bioactivation, is the conversion of genotoxic benzo-A-pyrene to the carcinogenic benzo-a-pyrene-diol-epoxides by the enzymatic action of CYP1A1 and CYP1B1 [48]. Other families of enzymes can also carry out a similar function in converting carcinogens to their active form, including sulfotransferase. Sulfotransferase family cytosolic 1B member 1 (SULT1B1) converts the genotoxic carcinogen aristolochic acid to its active form by the action of sulfotransferase enzymes specifically SULT1B1 [49].

9. *In vitro* carcinogenicity screening

The Ames test is a bacterial mutagenicity assay, which is designed to be able to detect a chemical's ability to induce DNA damage that leads to gene mutations. The Ames test was first developed by the work of Bruce Ames, where he attempted to detect chemical mutagens with the use of bacteria [50]. This now well established assay works with the use of different strains of Salmonella that have mutations in genes involved in histidine synthesis, this causes the bacteria to be unable to grow [51]. The principle of the Ames test is based on whether a chemical can induce mutations that can cause the bacteria to again produce histidine which would then allow bacterial growth. To allow for the detection of various mutagens that function by different mechanisms different strains of salmonella are used that have varying mutations in the histidine operon [51]. Over the years the Ames test has undergone a number of modifications from the original method [52]. The most significant improvement was the incorporation of rat liver microsomes, which allowed for the screening of the original compound undergoing testing and any potentially carcinogenic metabolites that could be produced [53]. In more recent years human liver S9 microsomal fractions have been utilised to try and improve the ability to detect carcinogens in humans. The main limitation of the Ames test still remains, which is *Salmonella typhimurium* being a prokaryote, however it is still useful as an initial carcinogenic screen.

Other *in vitro* screens for identifying carcinogens are collectively called cell transformation assays (CTAs). CTAs were first developed in the 1960s, in a study by Berwald et al. they showed that a carcinogenic hydrocarbon (Benzo-A-pyrene) was able to cause a transformation from normal cells to tumour cells [54]. The three main assays used nowadays are the BALB/c 3 t3 assay (mouse embryo cells), the Syrian hamster embryo cells (SHE) assay and C3H10T1/2 assay (pluripotent stem cells) [55]. The Organisation for Economic Co-operation and Development (OECD) carried out a very comprehensive review of the BALB/c 3T3, SHE and C3H10T1/2 assays. Each of the assays were assessed based on a number of criteria including sensitivity, specificity and predictivity. The C3H10T1/2 assay had the highest predictivity percentage of human carcinogens at 95%, this was followed by SHE and BALB/c 3T3 assays that had predictivity of 88 and 77% respectively [56]. Being able to predict the carcinogenicity of non-genotoxic carcinogens has been a major problem in carcinogenic screening, this has been somewhat overcome with the use of CTAs as the transformation of cells occurs with both genotoxic and non-genotoxic carcinogens [57]. As well as being used as screens for carcinogens CTAs are also used in investigating tumour initiation, evaluating classes of chemicals and establishing mechanism of action of compounds [55].

In 2006, the EU introduced the registration, evaluation, authorisation and restriction of chemicals (REACH) initiative. The implementation of these policies highlights the needs for an improved protection of human and environmental health and safety by the identification of potentially dangerous chemicals and their exact mechanisms of hazardness. These regulations have been phased in gradually over an 11 year period since their inception [58]. This has led to much stricter rules and regulation being put in place for the chemical industry and the need for improved carcinogenicity screening methods. Although very useful in predicting carcinogenic potential, the limitations of *in vitro* testing methods must also be recognised. In a study by Walmsley et al. they highlight the challenges involved in *in vitro* screens where non-carcinogens can sometimes be determined as carcinogens and the difficulties this can cause [59].

10. Animal models based carcinogenicity screening

A 2 year rodent bioassay is widely used in carcinogenicity risk assessment. The goal of this screening method is to be able to predict potential carcinogenicity, while also characterising any potential tumour development. Before the 2-year study commences either or both 14 or 90 day pre-chronic study must be completed to establish maximum tolerated doses [60]. *The National Toxicology Programme* set out a protocol in 1976 that is still used today. This protocol involves the use of 50 animals per sex per group [61]. The testing system is categorised into acute, sub-chronic and chronic exposure and in some cases *in utero* exposure. The study concludes with a histological assessment to identify any potential carcinogenic related changes. Attempts have been made to improve on the traditional 2-year rodent method, one such suggestion by Cohen et al. proposed that the 2 year study should be replaced by an enhanced 13 week screen [62]. This study suggests a shorter more robust study is sufficient to predict carcinogenicity, thus reducing the number of animals used, as well as time and costs.

The proposed screening process involves a tiered approach where the first step is to establish genotoxicity, estrogenic/immunosuppressive activity, this would then be followed by a multi dose response screen of the compounds effects on cell proliferation and overall toxicity. However, this shortened screen could fail to predict the carcinogenicity of a chemical where the effects take longer than 13-weeks to emerge. The main arguments against the use of the well-established 2-year rodent bioassay will always be whether this particular animal is suitable for predicting disease in humans and the issue of the unnecessary use of animal models. These limitations have been further highlighted with the EU's commitment to 'reduce, refine and replace animal models' [63].

Due to the kidneys function as a blood filtration system, it allows for the exposure and accumulation of potentially carcinogenic substances, leaving the kidneys to be susceptible to the development of various forms of renal carcinomas. For this reason there is an ever increasing need to improve screening methods that are capable of detecting carcinogens particularly those known to induce the development of kidney cancers.

Acknowledgements

This work was supported by Science Foundation Ireland.

Author details

Michael Higgins, Ismael Obaidi and Tara McMorrow*

*Address all correspondence to: tara.mcmorrow@ucd.ie

School of Biomolecular and Biomedical Sciences, Conway Institute, University College Dublin, Dublin, Ireland

References

[1] Siegel RL, Miller KD, Jemal A. Cancer statistics, 2016. CA: A Cancer Journal for Clinicians. 2016;**66**(1):7-30

[2] Koul H et al. Molecular aspects of renal cell carcinoma: A review. American Journal of Cancer Research. 2011;**1**(2):240-254

[3] Znaor A, Lortet-Tieulent J, Laversanne M, Jemal A, Bray F. International variations and trends in renal cell carcinoma incidence and mortality. European Urology. March 2015;**67**(3):519-530

[4] Jonasch E, Gao JJ, Rathmell WK. Renal cell carcinoma. BMJ (British Medical Journal). 2014;**349**:g4797

[5] Cancer Facts & Figures 2013. American Cancer Society; 2013

[6] Cairns P. Renal cell carcinoma. Cancer Biomarkers. 2011;**9**(1-6):461-473

[7] Muglia VF, Prando A. Renal cell carcinoma: Histological classification and correlation with imaging findings. Radiologia Brasileira; **48**(3):166-174

[8] Su D et al. Renal cell carcinoma: molecular biology and targeted therapy. Current Opinion in Oncology; **26**(3):321-327

[9] Gnarra JR et al. Mutations of the VHL tumour suppressor gene in renal carcinoma. Nature Genetics. 1994;**7**(1):85-90

[10] Brugarolas J. Molecular genetics of clear-cell renal cell carcinoma. Journal of Clinical Oncology; **32**(18):1968-1976

[11] Guo HF et al. The PI3K/AKT pathway and renal cell carcinoma. Journal of Genetics and Genomics. 2015;**42**(7):343-353

[12] Vera-Badillo FE, Conde E, Duran I. Chromophobe renal cell carcinoma: A review of an uncommon entity. International Journal of Urology; **19**(10):894-900

[13] Amin MB et al. Chromophobe renal cell carcinoma: Histomorphologic characteristics and evaluation of conventional pathologic prognostic parameters in 145 cases. The American Journal of Surgical Pathology. 2008;**32**(12):1822-1834

[14] Dason S et al. Management of renal collecting duct carcinoma: A systematic review and the McMaster experience. Current Oncology; **20**(3):e223-e232

[15] Kell S. Renal cell carcinoma: Treatment options. British Journal of Nursing. 2011;**20**(9): 536-539

[16] Krabbe LM et al. Surgical management of metastatic renal cell carcinoma in the era of targeted therapies. World Journal of Urology; **32**(3):615-622

[17] Huang WC et al. Chronic kidney disease after nephrectomy in patients with renal cortical tumours: A retrospective cohort study. The Lancet Oncology. 2006;**7**(9):735-740

[18] Hutson TE. Renal cell carcinoma: Diagnosis and treatment, 1994-2003. Proceedings (Baylor University Medical Center). 2005;**18**(4):337-340

[19] Klatte T et al. Understanding the natural biology of kidney cancer: Implications for targeted cancer therapy. Revista de Urología. 2007;**9**(2):47-56

[20] Zarogoulidis P et al. mTOR pathway: A current, up-to-date mini-review (review). Oncology Letters; **8**(6):2367-2370

[21] Battelli C, Cho DC. mTOR inhibitors in renal cell carcinoma. Therapy; **8**(4):359-367

[22] IARC. IARC monographs of the evaluation of carcinogenic risks to humans. IARC Monograph. 25 June 2012;**100A**:1

[23] Baba AI, Câtoi C. Comparative Oncology. 2007

[24] Paolini M et al. Beta-carotene: A cancer chemopreventive agent or a co-carcinogen? Mutation Research. 2003;**543**(3):195-200

[25] Lee SJ et al. Distinguishing between genotoxic and non-genotoxic hepatocarcinogens by gene expression profiling and bioinformatic pathway analysis. Scientific Reports. 2013;**3**:2783

[26] Lima BS, Van der Laan JW. Mechanisms of nongenotoxic carcinogenesis and assessment of the human hazard. Regulatory Toxicology and Pharmacology. 2000;**32**(2):135-143

[27] van Delft JHM et al. Discrimination of genotoxic from non-genotoxic carcinogens by gene expression profiling (vol 25, pg 1265, 2004). Carcinogenesis. 2005;**26**(2):511-511

[28] Lee YS et al. Induction of oh8Gua glycosylase in rat kidneys by potassium bromate (KBrO3), a renal oxidative carcinogen. Mutation Research. 1996;**364**(3):227-233

[29] Moller L, Zeisig M. DNA adduct formation after oral administration of 2-nitrofluorene and N-acetyl-2-aminofluorene, analyzed by 32P-TLC and 32P-HPLC. Carcinogenesis. 1993;**14**(1):53-59

[30] Ruggeri B et al. Benzo[a]pyrene-induced murine skin tumors exhibit frequent and characteristic G to T mutations in the p53 gene. Proceedings of the National Academy of Sciences of the United States of America. 1993;**90**(3):1013-1017

[31] Grollman AP. Aristolochic acid nephropathy: Harbinger of a global iatrogenic disease. Environmental and Molecular Mutagenesis. 2013;**54**(1):1-7

[32] Arison RN, Feudale EL. Induction of renal tumour by streptozotocin in rats. Nature. 1967;**214**(5094):1254-1255

[33] Robbiano L et al. DNA damage induced by seven N-nitroso compounds in primary cultures of human and rat kidney cells. Mutation Research. 1996;**368**(1):41-47

[34] Majeed S et al. Aflatoxins and ochratoxin A contamination in rice, corn and corn products from Punjab, Pakistan. Journal of Cereal Science. 2013;**58**(3):446-450

[35] Duris D et al. Ochratoxin A contamination of coffee batches from Kenya in relation to cultivation methods and post-harvest processing treatments. Food Additives and Contaminants. Part A, Chemistry Analysis Control Exposure & Risk Assessment. 2010;**27**(6):836-841

[36] Clark HA, Snedeker SM. Ochratoxin A: Its cancer risk and potential for exposure. Journal of Toxicology and Environmental Health. Part B, Critical Reviews. 2006;**9**(3):265-296

[37] Grosse Y et al. Formation of Ochratoxin-A metabolites and DNA-adducts in monkey kidney-cells. Chemico-Biological Interactions. 1995;**95**(1-2):175-187

[38] Mally A, Dekant W. DNA adduct formation by ochratoxin A: Review of the available evidence. Food Additives and Contaminants. Part A, Chemistry Analysis Control Exposure & Risk Assessment. 2005;**22**:65-74

[39] Mantle PG et al. Structures of covalent adducts between DNA and ochratoxin A: A new factor in debate about genotoxicity and human risk assessment. Chemical Research in Toxicology. 2010;**23**(1):89-98

[40] Schaaf GJ et al. The role of oxidative stress in the ochratoxin A-mediated toxicity in proximal tubular cells. Biochimica et Biophysica Acta-Molecular Basis of Disease. 2002; **1588**(2):149-158

[41] NTP toxicology and carcinogenesis studies of monuron (CAS No. 150-68-5) in F344/N rats and B6C3F1 mice (feed studies). National Toxicology Program Technical Report Series. 1988;**266**:1-166

[42] Bloch KM et al. Transcriptomic alterations induced by monuron in rat and human renal proximal tubule cells in vitro and comparison to rat renal-cortex in vivo. Toxicology Research. 2015;**4**(2):423-431

[43] Elcombe CR et al. Prediction of rodent nongenotoxic carcinogenesis: Evaluation of biochemical and tissue changes in rodents following exposure to nine nongenotoxic NTP carcinogens. Environmental Health Perspectives. 2002;**110**(4):363-375

[44] Ishidate M. Data Book of Chromosomal Aberration Test In vitro. New York: Elsevier; 1987. pp. 49-50

[45] EPA. Chlorothalonil Reregistration Eligibility Decision Team. EPA 738-R-99-004. 1999

[46] Radford R et al. Mechanisms of chemical carcinogenesis in the kidneys. International Journal of Molecular Sciences. 2013;**14**(10):19416-19433

[47] Ioannides C, Lewis DFV. Cytochromes P450 in the bioactivation of chemicals. Current Topics in Medicinal Chemistry. 2004;**4**(16):1767-1788

[48] Uppstad H et al. Importance of CYP1A1 and CYP1B1 in bioactivation of benzo[a]pyrene in human lung cell lines. Toxicology Letters. 2010;**192**(2):221-228

[49] Sidorenko VS et al. Bioactivation of the human carcinogen aristolochic acid. Carcinogenesis. 2014;**35**(8):1814-1822

[50] McCann J, Ames BN. Discussion paper: The detection of mutagenic metabolites of carcinogens in urine with the salmonella/microsome test. Annals of the New York Academy of Sciences. 1975;**269**:21-25

[51] Mortelmans K, Zeiger E. The Ames Salmonella/microsome mutagenicity assay. Mutation Research, Fundamental and Molecular Mechanisms of Mutagenesis. 2000;**455**(1-2):29-60

[52] Maron DM, Ames BN. Revised methods for the Salmonella mutagenicity test. Mutation Research. 1983;**113**(3-4):173-215

[53] Malling HV. Mutagenic activation of dimethylnitrosamine and diethyl-nitrosamine in the host-mediated assay and the microsomal system. Mutation Research. 1974;**26**(6):465-472

[54] Berwald Y, Sachs L. In vitro transformation of normal cells to tumor cells by carcinogenic hydrocarbons. Journal of the National Cancer Institute. 1965;**35**(4):641-661

[55] Creton S et al. Cell transformation assays for prediction of carcinogenic potential: State of the science and future research needs. Mutagenesis; **27**(1):93-101

[56] Vasseur P, Lasne C. OECD Detailed Review Paper (DRP) number 31 on "Cell Transformation Assays for Detection of Chemical Carcinogens": Main results and conclusions. Mutation Research; **744**(1):8-11

[57] Ohmori K et al. An assay method for the prediction of tumor promoting potential of chemicals by the use of Bhas 42 cells. Mutation Research. 2004;**557**(2):191-202

[58] C1 Regulation (EC) No 1907/2006 of The European Parliament and of Council Regulation 2006. 1907/2006

[59] Walmsley RM, Billinton N. How accurate is in vitro prediction of carcinogenicity? British Journal of Pharmacology. 2011;**162**(6):1250-1258

[60] Marone PA, Hall WC, Hayes AW. Reassessing the two-year rodent carcinogenicity bioassay: A review of the applicability to human risk and current perspectives. Regulatory Toxicology and Pharmacology. 2014;**68**(1):108-118

[61] NTP. Guidelines for Carcinogen Bioassay in Small Rodents. National Cancer Institute: Carcinogenesis 1976. Technical Report Series No. 1

[62] Cohen SM. An enhanced 13-week bioassay: An alternative to the 2-year bioassay to screen for human carcinogenesis. Experimental and Toxicologic Pathology. 2010;**62**(5):497-502

[63] Parliament E. Directive 2010/63/EU of The European Parliament and of The Council of 22 September 2010 on the Protection of Animals used for Scientific Purposes. L 276/33, 2010

Chapter 3

Increased Air Pollution Causing Cancers and Its Rapid Online Monitoring

Jianhai Sun, Jinhua Liu, Chunxiu Liu, Yanni Zhang,
Xiaofeng Zhu, Jingjing Zhang and Zhanwu Ning

Additional information is available at the end of the chapter

http://dx.doi.org/10.5772/intechopen.71366

Abstract

Pollution of indoor and outdoor air has considerably been taken attention abroad as an important environmental problem, and there is sufficient evidence that exposure to outdoor air pollution causes lung cancer and other cancers. Therefore, the current situation of air pollution will be deeply discussed, and a portable environmental gas monitor integrated by a variety of highly sensitive sensors will be developed for rapidly monitoring air pollution, which is able to provide scientific data for environmental pollution control. By this way, human beings are able to be far away from cancer caused by environmental pollution and its suffering.

Keywords: air pollution, portable environmental gas monitor, volatile organic compounds, toxic gases, metal oxide sensor, particulate matters, photoionization detector

1. Introduction

Cancer is caused by changes in certain genes that alter the function of our cells. Some of these genetic changes occur naturally when DNA is replicated during the process of cell division. But others are the result of DNA damage caused by environmental exposure, and these exposures include toxic and harmful gases, repairable dust, chemicals, and radiation.

The air we breathe has been contaminated with a mixture of carcinogens [1–3]. We now know that outdoor or indoor air pollution has been acted as a major health risk [1–11] but also a leading environmental cause of cancer deaths. The risk of developing lung cancer is significantly increased in people exposed to air pollution. Air pollution is a gas (or a liquid or solid

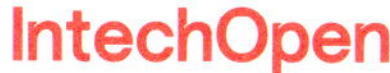

dispersed through ordinary air) released with a big-enough quantity to harm health of people or other animals, kill plants or stop them growing properly, damage or disrupt some other aspect of the environment (such as making buildings crumble), or cause some other kind of nuisance (reduced visibility, perhaps, or an unpleasant odor). Air pollution is predominantly caused by automobile exhaust, industrial and agricultural emissions, construction dust, chemical leakage, residential heating and cooking, as well as some pollution accidents (such as factory explosion, toxic runway and playground, etc.). It is uncertain to what degree air pollution contributes to cancer, but according to the largest study to date, more than 10% of lung cancers may be caused by air pollution. Moreover, experts have identified other ills caused by the air pollution, including an increased risk of asthma and heart disease.

It is generally known that a variety of harmful gases will be present in the air when air pollution occurs, and if the harmful gases reached a high enough concentration, the air becomes very harmful to human health. When we talk about the harmful gases, there are dozens of different pollution gases in the air. In practice, about several different substances cause most concern, and these harmful gases are mainly sulfur dioxide, carbon monoxide, carbon dioxide, nitrogen oxides, volatile organic compounds (VOCs), ozone [12, 13], particulates [13–18], and so on. Therefore, let us talk about the sources of these toxic gases and their major dangers.

Carbon monoxide (CO): CO is mainly come from the incomplete combustion of C, such as automobile exhaust, coal combustion (especially coal-fired power plants and coal-fired supply heating system, etc.), fuel-burning appliance, and so on. It is well known that CO with high concentrations can directly cause death.

Carbon dioxide (CO_2): CO_2 is one of basic component of the atmosphere, just as the N_2 and O_2, and this gas is central to everyday life and is not normally considered as a pollutant. We all produce it when we breathe out, and plants such as crops and trees need to "breathe" it in to grow. However, CO_2 with high concentrations can also directly cause suffocation or even death.

Sulfur dioxide: coal, petroleum, and other fuels are often impure and contain sulfur as well as organic compounds. When sulfur burns with oxygen from the air, sulfur dioxide (SO_2) is produced. In the atmosphere, sulfur dioxide can be oxidized to sulfuric acid fog or sulfate aerosol, which is an important precursor of environmental acidification. There is a potential impact on the human body when the concentration of sulfur dioxide in the atmosphere is above 0.5 ppm, most people will begin to feel stimulated when the concentration of SO_2 is over 1 ppm, and people suffer from ulcers and pulmonary edema and even death by asphyxiation when the concentration is over 400 ppm. Sulfur dioxide has synergistic effects with soot in the atmosphere. When the concentration of sulfur dioxide in the atmosphere is 0.21 ppm, the concentration of smoke and dust is greater than 0.3 mg/l, the incidence of respiratory diseases can be increased, and the condition of the patients with chronic diseases will deteriorate rapidly. Such as the London smog event, Maas Valley events, Donora smog, and other events were all caused by this synergistic effect.

Nitrogen oxides: nitrogen dioxide (NO_2) and nitrogen oxide (NO) are pollutants produced as an indirect result of combustion when nitrogen and oxygen from the air react together.

Nitrogen oxide pollution comes from automobile exhaust and power plants and plays an important role in the formation of acid rain, ozone, and smog. Nitrogen oxides are also "indirect greenhouse gases" because they contribute to global warming by producing ozone. Nitrogen oxides mainly damage the respiratory tract, and if people are living in this environment for a long time, people may suffer from delayed pulmonary edema and adult respiratory distress syndrome.

Volatile organic compounds (VOCs): these carbon-based (organic) chemicals evaporate easily at ordinary temperatures and pressures, so they readily become gases. That's precisely why they are used as solvents in many different household chemicals such as paints, waxes, and varnishes. Indoor VOCs which are greatly harmful emit mainly from building and building fitment materials. Unfortunately, VOCs are greatly harmful and have long-term effects on human health, and they also play a role in the formation of ozone and smog. Therefore, it is necessary to investigate emission of VOCs and its controlling method.

Particulates: the particles can be deposited in the respiratory tract, lung, and other parts due to small size. The smaller the particle size of the PM is, the deeper the PM enters into the respiratory tract. It is well known that the PM with 10 μm diameter is deposited in the upper respiratory tract, the PM with 5 μm diameter can enter into the deep part of the respiratory tract, and the PM with diameter less than 2 μm can be easily penetrated deep into bronchioles and alveoli, which was easy to cause cancer and other diseases. Therefore, it is of great significance to develop a rapid on-site detection technique for inhalable particles, which will be very conducive to the understanding of the formation mechanism of fog and haze. In cities, most particulates come from traffic fumes.

Ozone: some of the ozone near the ground comes from the upper layer of ozone, and some of the ozone comes from the soil, lightning, biological emissions, etc. These can be classified as "natural sources", already in nature. The main cause of ozone pollution is "anthropogenic sources". Coal, vehicle exhaust, petrochemical, and other pollutants (for example, NOx (nitrogen oxides)) will produce ozone and other NOx, which is called the two photochemical reaction. Studies have shown that only 23% total ozone pollution occurred each year in the near ground layer comes from the nature's own transport and as high as 48% total ozone comes from the photochemical reaction from NOx and other pollutants. It can be said that the concentration of ozone in urban areas depends mainly on the emission of motor vehicles exhaust. Ozone can cause great harm to the human body: ozone can damage lung function, stimulate respiratory tract, cause airway reaction, increase airway inflammation, and aggravate asthma. High levels of persistent ozone pollution may cause watering eyes, eye pain, headaches, and other symptoms, which can affect the respiratory and cardiovascular systems.

In this chapter, a portable gas monitor fabricated for rapidly monitoring air pollution was developed, and the systems consists of the following modules: an automated sampling device, multisensors-integrated sensing system, a signal acquisition, processing and display system, and a power supply. Finally, the proposed systems were used to monitor air pollution in various environmental sites, such as industrial chemical plan, pesticide plants, printing and dyeing plants, pesticide plants, and so on. These environmental pollution data will be provided to the local environmental monitoring department, and these data are very important for the purification and treatment of the environment, so that we are able to avoid the high-risk air pollution and the cancers caused by air pollution.

2. Experimental details

2.1. The schematic of the minienvironmental gas system

In order to effectively monitor toxic and harmful gas in the air, a multisensor integrated into the portable system is proposed, and its structure diagram was shown in **Figure 1**. The system mainly includes the following parts: (1) automatic injection system, (2) purification unit for sample, (3) gas sensing unit (4), signal acquisition, output, and display unit, and (5) power supply. The sampling section mainly includes a sampling pipe and a sampling pump, in which the sampling pipe was inserted into pollutant source or possible leakage spots, and then, the sample was pumped and transported into the purification unit. The purification unit consists of sample filtration and sample drying, by which the particulate matters are filtered through a filter membrane with pore size of 0.22 μm made by PTFE material, and at the same time, moisture was absorbed and removed by the purifying material packed in chamber of the purification unit. After the sample has been purified, the sample was then transported into the sensor unit for target identification and concentration identification. The sensing unit is the brain of the whole system, which consists of a variety of highly sensitive sensors, and each sensor can accurately identify a component and detect its concentration. Moreover, in the system, we can choose sensor combinations according to different application areas (different kinds of harmful gas) because the environmental gases contain some of the harmful gases, such as O_3, H_2S, CO, NO_2, NH_3, SO_2, formaldehyde, VOCs, and NO. Therefore, according to the different applications, some different high sensitive sensors were integrated into the system, such as mini PID sensor, H_2S sensor, SO_2 sensor, NO sensor, NO_2 sensor, NH_3 sensor, O_3 sensor, and so on. The signal processing system mainly includes signal acquisition, processing, transmission, and display. An output signal proportional to the concentration was obtained from the sensor, after the signal was processed by high-accurate AD converter

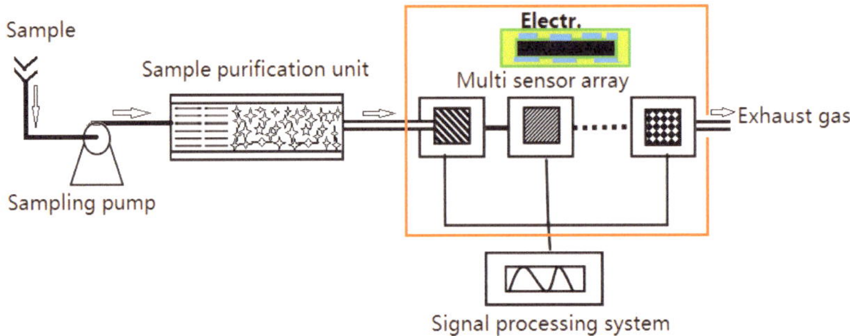

Figure 1. Schematic diagram of the portable gas monitor.

and MCU, the types and concentrations of this contaminated gas were displayed by a mini PC or liquid crystal display (LCD).

2.2. Highly sensitive sensors

2.2.1. High performance of mini PID

A photoionization detector (PID) uses an ultraviolet (UV) light source to ionize gas molecules to positive and negative ions that can be easily measured with a detector. The PID is commonly employed in the detection of volatile organic compounds (VOCs) such as alkanes, alkenes, oxygenated hydrocarbons, and halogenated hydrocarbons, etc. VOCs mainly come from the following aspects: industrial stationary source, vehicle exhaust emission source, and daily life source. The PID detectors are able to detect traces gas with concentration of ppb level and provide an instant reading indicating whether gas is present, which makes PID sensors useful in go/no-go situations, where personnel are unsure of what threats they face.

In this work, a mini PID detector has been developed, which can be used to detect volatile organic compounds in the environment with high sensitivity. In order to improve sensitivity of the PID, a little ionization chamber with volume of 10 μl, which was made of polytetrafluoroethylene (PTFE), was proposed. **Figure 2(a)** shows a side view of the ionization chamber and the fabricated mini PID. **Figure 2(b)** indicates photo of the fabricated PID. The characteristic of the fabricated PID was the little volume of the ionization chamber, dramatically reducing velocity of carrier gas (velocity of carrier gas was able to be reduced to less than 10 ml/min). The proposed PID demonstrated high-detection performance (refer to **Table 1**) by effectively reducing background noises, external electromagnetic interferences, and the ionization chamber volume.

In this work, in order to accurately detect the concentration of the VOCs come from pollution source, the fabricated PID was integrated into the monitoring system.

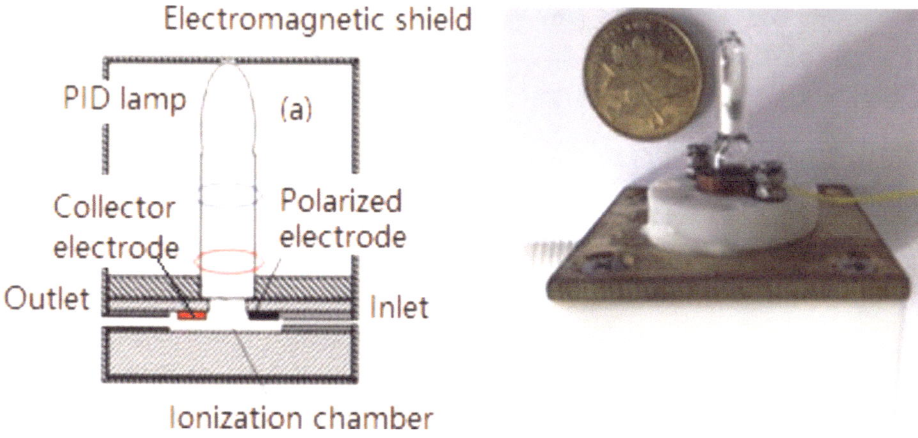

Figure 2. (a) Schematic of the fabricated mini PID, (b) photo of the fabricated PID.

Detection limit (for benzene)	1 ppb
Relative standard deviation (RSD)	0.5%
Baseline drift	1.0×10^{-13} A/30 min
Background noise	Less than 1.0×10^{-13} A
Linear range (for benzene)	10^5

Table 1. A summarized performance of the fabricated mini PID.

2.2.2. *High sensitivity sensors*

In order to effectively monitor these environmental harmful gases (such as O_3, H_2S, CO, NO_2, NH_3, SO_2, formaldehyde, VOCs, NO and so on), some highly sensitive sensors were selected to monitor these harmful gases, and the response characteristics of each sensor will be described as follows.

The H_2S sensor based on electrochemical principles is able to detect trace concentrations below 10 ppb, and **Figure 3** shows the responses to 200 ppb sample gases. The data indicate that the sensor has high resolution and good linearity, which is suitable for the analysis of trace gases in the environment.

The SO_2, NO, and O_3 sensor also based on electrochemical principles were able to detect trace concentrations, and **Figures 4–6** show the responses to sample gases. These experiment results show that these sensors have high sensitivity and can be used to detect various pollution sources in ambient air.

The formaldehyde sensor responds to formaldehyde that are electrochemically active, and the bias voltage of +300 mV is optimum for formaldehyde; however, the sensor also responds to other VOCs under other bias voltage. If the formaldehyde needs to be detected with high precision, TVOCs needs to be tested at once and then eliminate its impact. **Figure 7** shows the response of 3.8 ppm formaldehyde using the sensor.

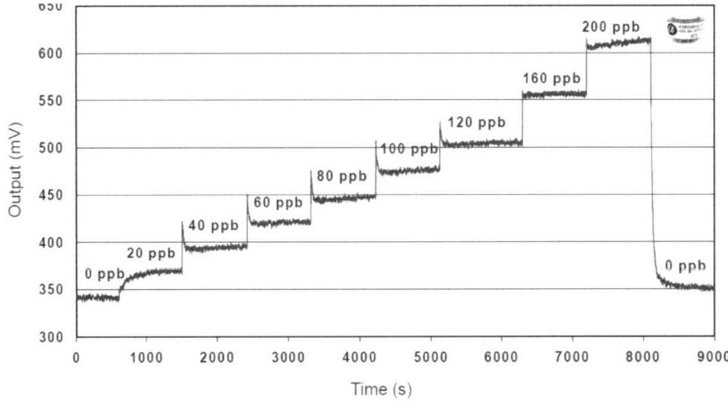

Figure 3. Response to 200 ppb H_2S using the H_2S sensor.

http://dx.doi.org/10.5772/intechopen.71366

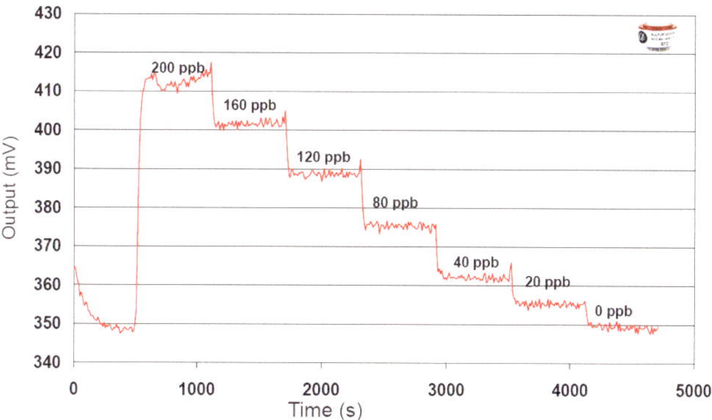

Figure 4. Response to 200 ppb SO_2 using the SO_2 sensor.

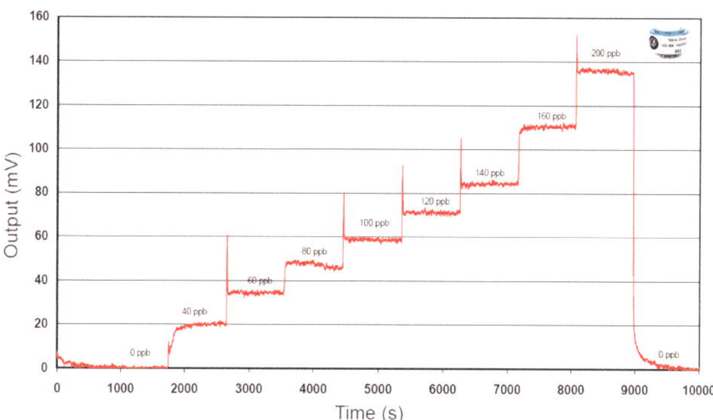

Figure 5. Response to 200 ppb NO using the NO sensor.

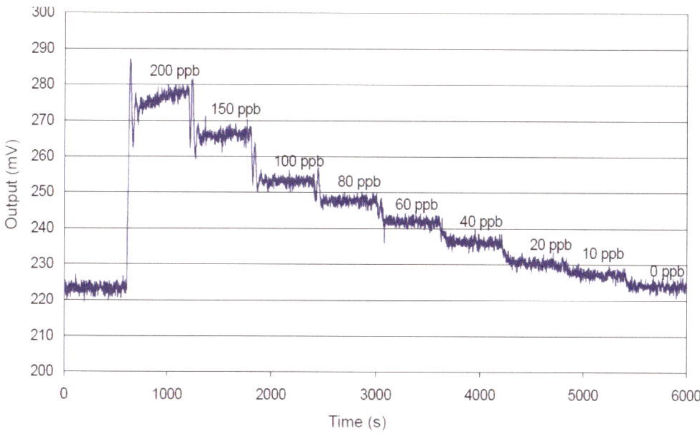

Figure 6. Response to 200 ppb O_3 using the O_3 sensor.

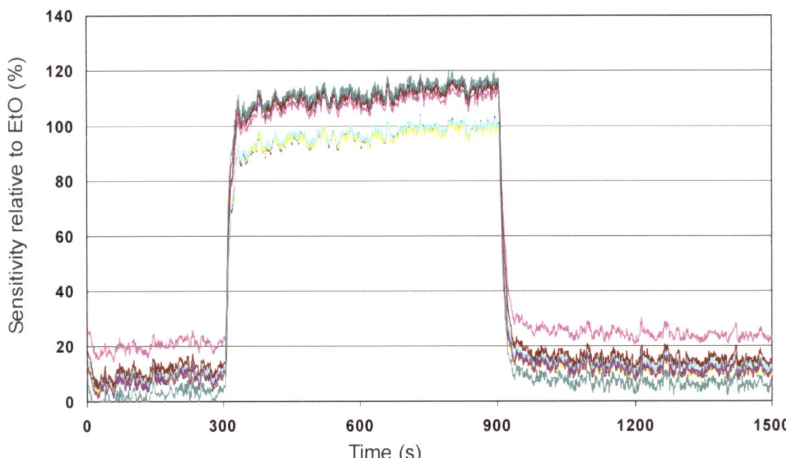

Figure 7. The response of 3.8 ppm formaldehyde.

Because of the basic principle of NDIR gas sensors, only the gas with asymmetric molecular structure can absorb strong infrared rays. Therefore, NDIR gas sensors can only measure SO_2, NO, CO_2, CO, CH_4, and other molecules with asymmetric molecular structure. For O_2, H_2, N_2, and other molecules with symmetrical molecular structure, the NDIR is incapable of action.

NDIR detectors are the industry standard method of measuring the concentration of carbon oxides (CO and CO_2). Each constituent gas in a sample will absorb some infrared at a particular frequency (**Figure 8** is the infrared absorption spectrum of CO_2). By shining an infrared beam through a sample chamber containing CO_2 and measuring the amount of infrared absorbed by the sample, the volumetric concentration of CO_2 in the sample can be reported. **Figure 9** shows the schematic diagram of the NDIR detector. In this work, a NDIR detector (Prime 2, purchased from Clairair Ltd.) was integrated for detecting the concentration of CO_2.

In this work, a microfabricated metal oxide (MOX) detector based on SnO/SnO_2/Au nanocomposite sensitive material was used to detect the CO gas. In order to increase conductivity of the sensitive material, SnO-doped sensitive material was proposed because of the low conductivity of SnO_2, which was able to greatly increase the activity of SnO_2 sensitive layer. The sensitive film (nano-metric thickness) was fabricated, and the process was defined as follows, and a schematic representation of the whole structure is depicted in **Figure 10**.

First of all, a layer of SnO and SnO_2 thin film deposited over the hotplate surface has been carried out by sputtering through a modified rheotaxial growth and thermal oxidation technique, and the thickness of the SnO and SnO_2 thin film was 50 nm and 150 nm, respectively. Then, an extremely thin Au film with thickness of 5 nm was deposited over its surface to act as a catalyst and consequently increase SnO_2 film selectivity. Finally, the release process (or suspension process) of the supported beam was shown as follows. A layer of photoresist with

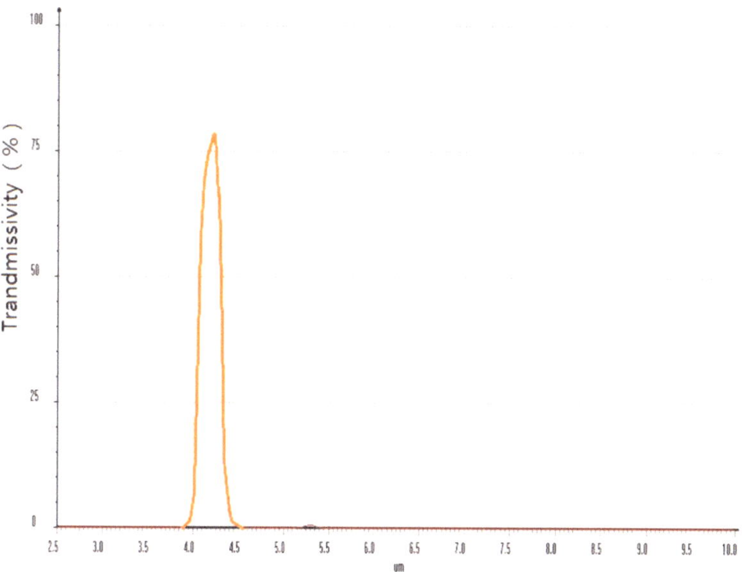

Figure 8. Infrared absorption spectrum of CO_2.

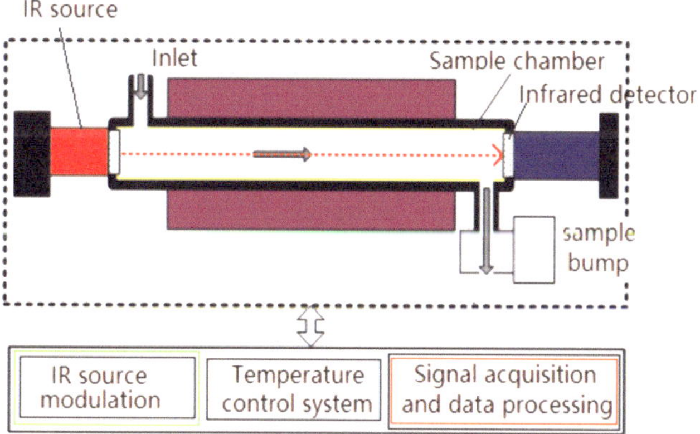

Figure 9. The schematic diagram of the NDIR detector.

thickness of 2 μm was coated and patterned as an etch mask for silicon nitride. After the two layers of the silicon nitride were etched by the reactive-ion etching (RIE) technology, a deep reactive-ion etching (DRIE) process was utilized to remove the diffusion of silicon in the micro channels. Then, the supported beam was released through a silicon etch (using 40 wt% KOH solution at 80°C for 70 min). The chip size (refer to **Figure 11**) is 8 × 10 mm^2 with an active area (for each of the four sensors) of 1 × 4 mm^2, consisting of platinum resistor acting as heater. The sensor can detect CO with a detection limit of 0.1 ppm, and the resolution of the sensor can be less than 1 ppm.

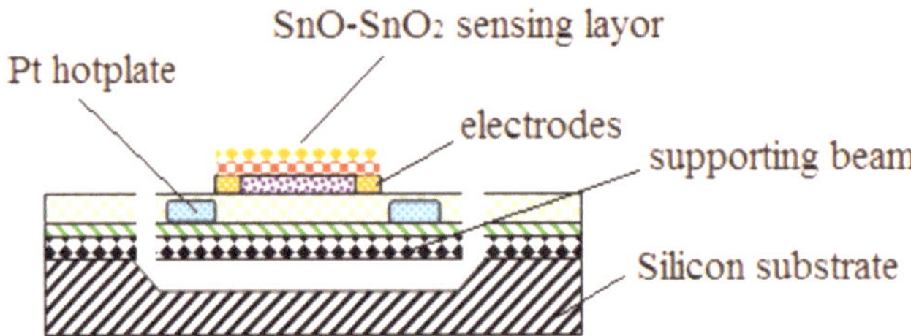

Figure 10. A schematic representation of the sensor.

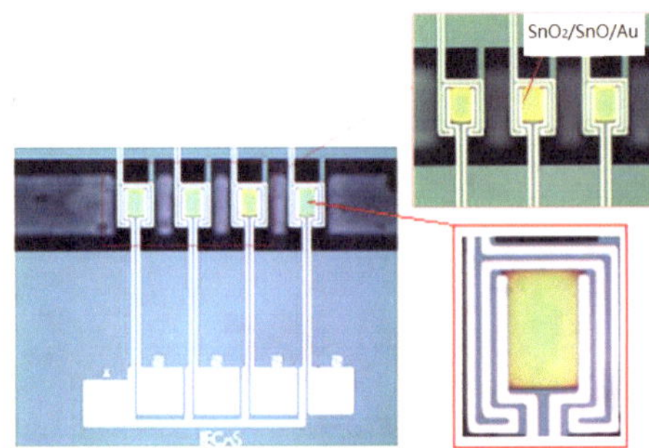

Figure 11. Photo of the MOX sensor based on $SnO/SnO_2/Au$ nanocomposite sensitive material.

The particles can be deposited in the respiratory tract, lung, and other parts due to small size. The smaller the particle size of the PM is, the deeper the PM enters into the respiratory tract. PM is the leading cause of pneumoconiosis. Therefore, PM is especially harmful to humans, and its formation and monitoring should be paid special attention. In this work, optical method was used to monitor the PM, which monitors the change of light intensity to determine the average concentration of PM. **Figure 12** shows the photo of the PM sensor and the working schematic diagram.

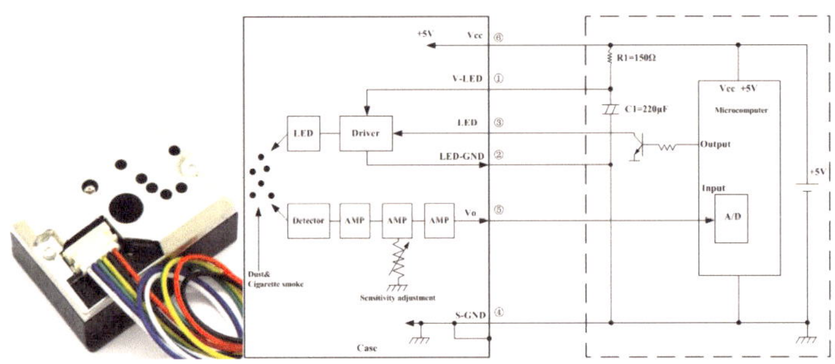

Figure 12. The PM sensor and the working schematic diagram.

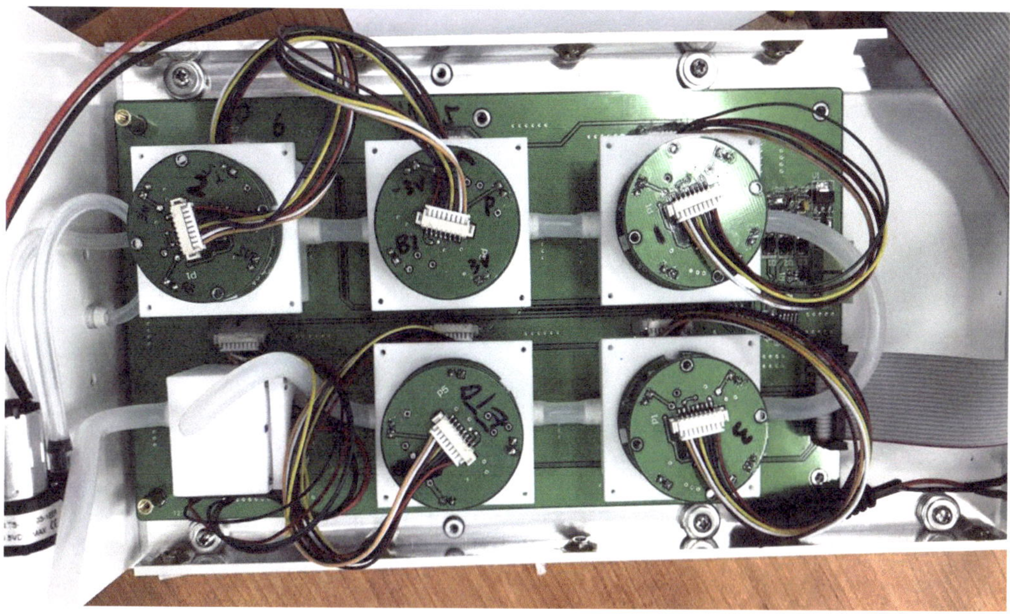

Figure 13. Portable environmental gas detection system.

2.3. Integration of monitoring system

In this work, the gas hoods using polytetrafluoroethylene (PTFE) for packaging these sensors were fabricated, and then these sensors were integrated into the system. **Figure 13** shows the photo of the portable system, in which the sample was transported by a mini pump and the power supply is a 12 V battery module. The data are processed through a high-resolution 24 bit AD (ADS1256) converter and displayed by a LCD. According to the application areas, we can easily change the sensor module.

3. Results and discussion

Air pollution has considerably been taken attention abroad as an important environmental problem, and there is sufficient evidence that exposure to air pollution causes lung cancer and other cancers. Therefore, it is necessary to develop highly sensitive systems to detect harmful gases. In this work, several different sensors were integrated into a portable system according to different application areas. For example, the proposed system integrated with TVOCs, H_2S, SO_2, CO, O_3, NO, CO_2, and formaldehyde sensor was used for monitoring pollution sources, such as the automobile coating industry, chemical processing industry, furniture manufacturing, oil refining, and chemical industry.

We selected a garage to monitor air pollution, it is well known that a lot of paint, gasoline, and lubricating oil was used at work, and a large amount of exhaust gas is emitted from the

	#1	#2	#3	#4	#5
TVOC (ppm)	5.524	5.461	5.556	5.270	5.353
H_2S (ppm)	0.564	0.556	0.578	0.489	0.486
SO_2 (ppm)	0.802	0.813	0.882	0.916	0.925
CO (ppm)	0.135	0.118	0.167	0.185	0.201
CO_2 (ppm)	578	586	592	597	620
O_3 (ppm)	0.225	0.186	0.175	0.216	0.228
NO (ppm)	0.102	0.125	0.118	0.102	0.128
Formaldehyde	1.068	1.025	1.086	1.164	1.125
PM 2.5 (μg/m^3)	230	243	241	236	230

Table 2. The concentration of each component in the garage detected by the monitor.

automobile; therefore, the component of the air is complex. In this work, the air pollution was monitored continuously using the proposed system. The testing cycle is every hour and 5 times in a row. **Table 2** indicates the concentration of each component of the garage detected by the monitor.

As we can see from the monitoring data, the concentration of TVOC, SO_2, H_2S, formaldehyde, O_3, NO, and PM are higher than their national standard in the auto repair factory. Obviously, these harmful gases will be harmful to health of workers if they work in such a "high pollution" environment for a long time, which will bring serious diseases and even cancer. In order to protect the health of workers, the air pollution need to be on-site monitored with high sensitive; at the same time, the harmful gases also need to be removed till their concentrations are reduced to the normal allowed level, which the workers can freely breathe the air.

4. Conclusion

The existence of a number of toxic and harmful gases has greatly damaged people's health. Therefore, real-time and high-precision detection of these gases is the primary basis for effective prevention of this pollution source, and the purpose of the elimination of these harmful gases can finally be achieved only through this high-precision detection technology. So that people can be away from cancer and be free breathing the air in the clean and blue sky.

Acknowledgements

The authors greatly acknowledge the financial support from National Key Research and Development Program of China under grant numbers: 2016YFF02045 and 2016YFC07006. The authors also greatly acknowledge the financial support from the National Science Foundation of China under grant numbers: 11574219, 61774157, and 61176112.

Author details

Jianhai Sun[1]*, Jinhua Liu[2], Chunxiu Liu[1], Yanni Zhang[2], Xiaofeng Zhu[2], Jingjing Zhang[1] and Zhanwu Ning[2]

*Address all correspondence to: jhsun@mail.ie.ac.cn

1 State Key Laboratory of Transducer Technology, Institute of Electronics, Chinese Academy of Sciences, Beijing, China

2 Beijing Municipal Institute of Labour Protection, Beijing, China

References

[1] Pekkanen J, Peter A, Hoek G, et al. Particulate air pollution and risk of ST-segment depression during repeated submaximal exercise tests among subjects with coronary heart disease. Circulation. 2002;**106**:933-938

[2] Peters A, Dockery DW, Muller JE, Mittleman MA. Increased particulate air pollution and the triggering of myocardial infaction. Circulation. 2001;**103**:2810-2815

[3] Ibald-Mulli A, Stieber J, Wichmann H, et al. Effects of air pollution on blood pressure a population-based approach. American Journal of Public Health. 2001;**91**:571-577

[4] Suwa T, Hogg JC, Quinlan KB, et al. Particulate air pollution induces progression of atherosclerosis. Journal of the American College of Cardiology. 2002;**39**:935-942

[5] Gold DR, Litonjua A, Schwartz J, et al. Ambient pollution and heart rate variability. Circulation. 2000;**101**:1267-1273

[6] Pope CA, Verrier RL, Lovett EG, et al. Heart rate variability associated with particulate air pollution. American Heart Journal. 1999;**138**:890-899

[7] Magari SR, Hauser R, Schwartz J, et al. Association of heart rate variability with occupational and environmental exposure to particulate air pollution. Circulation. 2001;**104**:986-991

[8] Stone PH, Godleski JJ. First steps toward understanding the pathophysiology between air pollution and cardiac mortality. American Heart Journal. 1999;**138**:804-807

[9] Peters A, Liu E, Verrier RL, Schwartz J, et al. Air pollution and incidence of cardiac arrhythmia. Epidemiology. 2000;**11**:11-17

[10] Ross R. Mechanisms of disease: Atherosclerosis an inflammatory disease. The New England Journal of Medicine. 1999;**340**:115-126

[11] Schachinger V, Britten MB, Zeiher AM. Prognostic impact of coronary vasodilator dysfunction on adverse long-term outcome of coronary heart disease. Circulation. 2000;**101**:1899-1906

[12] Brook RD, Brook JR, Urch B, et al. Inhalation of fine particulate air pollution and ozone causes acute arterial vasoconstriction in healthy adults. Circulation. 2002;**105**:1534-1536

[13] Bouthillier L, Vincent R, Geogan P, et al. Acute effects of inhaled urban particles and ozone. The American Journal of Pathology. 1998;**153**:1-12

[14] Quillen JE, Rossen JD, Oskarsson HJ, et al. Acute effect of cigarette smoking on the coronary circulation: Constriction of epicardial and resistance vessels. Journal of the American College of Cardiology. 1993;**22**:642-649

[15] Goerre S, Staehli C, Shaw S, et al. Effect of cigarette smoking and nicotine on plasma endothelin-1 levels. Journal of Cardiovascular Pharmacology. 1995;**26**:S236-S238

[16] Otsuka R, Watanabe H, Hirata K, et al. Acute effects of passive smoking on the coronary circulation in healthy young adults. Journal of the American Medical Association. 2001;**286**:436-441

[17] Ikeda M, Watarai K, Suzuki M, et al. Mechanism of pathophysiological effects of diesel exhaust particles on endothelial cells. Environmental Toxicology and Pharmacology. 1998;**6**:117-123

[18] Ghio AJ, Kim C, Devlin RB. Concentrated ambient air particles induce mild pulmonary inflammation in healthy human volunteers. American Journal of Respiratory and Critical Care Medicine. 2000;**162**(3):981-988

Chapter 4

Cancer Causing Chemicals

Maher Soliman

Additional information is available at the end of the chapter

http://dx.doi.org/10.5772/intechopen.71560

Abstract

Carcinogens are substances that induce cancer by damaging the genome or through disruption of cellular metabolic processes. Some compounds interact directly with DNA, while others are activated to reactive molecules that can bind with DNA by covalent adducts causing mutations in genes crucial to biological processes. Cigarette smoke is by far the most important and notorious carcinogen. Cigarette smoke contains many carcinogenic substances including polycyclic aromatic hydrocarbons (PAHs), which are known to cause cancer. Nitrites, which are present in many foods, are converted into nitrous acid in the stomach and may then react with amines in food to produce nitrosamines, which are carcinogenic. Aflatoxins produced by Aspergillus flavus are promoter for hepatic cancer. Several cytotoxic drugs are carcinogens especially alkylating agents that interact with DNA. Individuals exposed to certain pesticides may be at risk to the development of certain cancers. Inorganic arsenic exposure has been suggested to be associated with the development of several cancers. Sufficient evidence indicated an association between dioxins and various cancers including soft tissue sarcoma, lymphoma and leukemia. Asbestos has been found to be significantly associated with lung cancer and mesothelioma.

Keywords: aflatoxins, cancer, carcinogens, carcinogenesis, chemicals, smoking

1. Introduction

Worldwide, cancer is a leading cause of mortality [1]. According to GLOBOCAN estimates, about 14.1 million new cancer cases and 8.2 million deaths occurred in 2012 worldwide [1]. The incidence and mortality rates of cancer differ between countries. However, over the last decades, the burden of cancer has shifted to less developed countries due to later stage of diagnosis and unavailability of treatment. Currently about 57% of cancer cases and 65% of cancer deaths occurs in less developed countries [1, 2]. The cancer profile also varies between countries. The incidence rates of prostate, colorectal, female breast and lung cancer are several

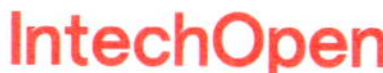

times higher in more developed countries compared with less developed countries. Liver, stomach, and cervical cancers are more frequent in less developed countries; these cancers are predominantly attributable to infection. However, lung cancer remains the leading cause of cancer death globally [1].

The burden of cancer is rising because of the aging of the population, and increasing exposure to established carcinogenic chemicals, viruses and radiations, as well as adoption of unhealthy lifestyle behaviors such as smoking, alcohol intake, overweight, and limited physical activity. Moreover, the success of screening programs and earlier detection of cancer have contributed to the rise of cancer problem [1, 2].

Carcinogens are substances which induce cancer, by damaging the genome or through disruption of cellular metabolic processes. Carcinogens have usually an insidious toxic effect rather than an acute toxic effect. Carcinogens could be either from synthetic chemicals or natural substances. Carcinogens can be classified as genotoxic or nongenotoxic agents according to mechanism of carcinogenesis. Genotoxins bind directly to DNA causing irreversible damage to the genome like polycyclic aromatic hydrocarbons (PAHs). Nongenotoxins do not directly affect DNA but could promote growth, like hormones and some organic compounds. Procarcinogens are not carcinogenic themselves, but turn into carcinogenic substances in the body, e.g. nitrates taken in the diet change into nitrosamines which is carcinogenic. Co-carcinogens are substances that promote the activity of other carcinogens in causing cancer but they are not carcinogenic on their own [3].

Chemical carcinogenesis was first described in 1775 by an eminent English physician and surgeon, Percivall Pott who observed the occurrence of cancer of the scrotum in a number of his patients who were chimney sweepers when they were young [3, 4]. Accordingly, Pott suggested that the occupation of these men as young boys and their exposure to large amounts of soot could be the causative agent of the cancer. One hundred years later, the high incidence of skin cancer among certain German workers was recognized to be associated to their exposure to coal tar, the chief constituent of the chimney sweeps' soot [5].

Only after 140 years of Dr. Pott's report of the association of epidermal cancer of the scrotum with the exposure to soot from the combustion of coal, the first experimental laboratory animal study on carcinogenesis was reported. In 1915, Yamagawa and Ichikawa first published a comprehensive paper describing the production of a malignant epidermal neoplasm by repeatedly applying crude coal tar to the ears of rabbits for a number of months [6]. Afterwards, several studies tried to define and isolate the causative carcinogenic substance from the crude tar. In 1930s, the first carcinogenic chemical compound, dibenz[a,h]anthracene was produced, followed by several polycyclic aromatic hydrocarbons (PAHs) were isolated from active crude tar fractions.

Since 1971, The International Agency for Research on Cancer (IARC) has evaluated more than 1000 agents, and has classified them into five groups as follows [7]:

- Group 1: Carcinogenic to humans (120 agents).
- Group 2A: Probably carcinogenic to humans (81 agents)

- Group 2B: Possibly carcinogenic to humans (299 agents)
- Group 3: Not classifiable as to its carcinogenicity to humans (502 agents)
- Group 4: Probably not carcinogenic to humans (1 agent)

2. Mechanisms of action of carcinogens

Carcinogenesis could be classified into four phases; initiation, promotion, progression and metastasis. Carcinogenic chemicals can initiate and/or promote this process by affecting the expression and activity of certain genes responsible for cell growth, differentiation, DNA repair, cell-cycle control, and apoptosis. Some compounds interact directly with DNA, while others are activated to reactive molecules that can bind with DNA by covalent adducts causing mutations in genes crucial to biological processes. Polycyclic aromatic hydrocarbons (PAHs) are known to cause cancer by forming covalent adducts with DNA, resulting in altered cell growth and repair [3].

Chemical carcinogens can target certain genes termed proto-oncogenes and tumor suppressor genes, which when become mutated, allow cells to grow without control like in breast, colon and lung cancers. Two well studied proto-oncogenes are MYC and RAS, which are responsible for regulation of the cell cycle and apoptosis. MYC function is involved in protein-protein interactions with various cellular factors such as in Burkitt's Lymphoma. RAS function as GTP-binding protein; important in signal transduction cascade such as in Pancreatic, Colorectal, Bladder Breast, Kidney, & Lung Neoplasms; Leukemia; Melanoma [8, 9]. Mutations in these genes can cause dysregulated cell division. The mutant proteins maintain their normal functions but are no longer under control of orders that regulate these processes. The products of RAS gene are essential components of kinase signaling pathways that regulate cell growth and differentiation. Mutations in RAS can be caused by organochlorine pesticide and exposure to arsenic [3].

One of the most well recognized tumor suppressor genes is p53 also known as TP53 or tumor protein (EC:2.7.1.37) is a gene that codes for a protein that regulates the cell cycle and hence functions as a tumor suppression. Under suboptimal conditions such as DNA damage, tumor suppressor genes produce products that inhibit cell division for growth. Mutations in p53 have been discovered in breast cancer and bronchial cancer exposed to organophosphorus pesticides and PAHs [10].

3. Some chemical carcinogens

3.1. Cigarette smoking

Cigarette smoking is the most important carcinogen. Cigarettes are the predominant type of tobacco product consumed in the world. Worldwide, more than 1 million cancer deaths are attributed to cigarette smoking annually. Cigarette smoking is the major cause of lung cancer.

Polycyclic aromatic hydrocarbons and the tobacco-specific nitrosamine 4-(methylnitrosamino)-1-(3-pyridyl)-1-butanone are likely to play major roles lung cancer induction [11].

Cigarette smoking is a major risk factor for cancers of oral cavity, oropharynx hypopharynx and Larynx, and the risk is greatly increased by alcohol consumption. Most cases of esophageal cancer, sinonasal and nasopharyngeal cancer, liver cancer, pancreatic cancer, stomach cancer, cervical squamous cell carcinoma, transitional cell carcinomas of the bladder, ureter, and renal pelvis and myeloid leukemia in adults are linked to cigarette smoking [12].

Laboratory studies clearly demonstrate that inhalation of cigarette smoke and topical application of cigarette smoke condensate (CSC) cause cancer in experimental animals. Studies identified the carcinogenic polycyclic aromatic hydrocarbons (PAHs) in cigarette smoke and showed that CSC has both carcinogenic and cocarcinogenic (tumor-promoting activity) effect. Tumors are not induced by the PAHs alone, using doses equivalent to their concentrations in CSC. However, carcinogenesis appears to depend on the composite interaction of the tumor initiators such as PAHs and tumor promoters [12].

Cigarette smoke contains more than 60 carcinogenic compounds that have been evaluated for carcinogenicity in laboratory animals, and 15 of them are considered as carcinogenic to humans. PAHs are a group of compounds produced from tobacco smoking. PAHs have a direct local carcinogenic effect. Benzo[a]pyrene, one of PAHs, has powerful carcinogenic activity to humans. Heterocyclic compounds are also combustion products and include nitrogen-containing analogues of PAHs such as furan, which is carcinogenic to liver [12].

N-nitrosamines are a large group of potent carcinogens. N-nitrosamines in cigarette smoke can induce lung tumors, tumors of the pancreas, nasal cavity, and liver and esophageal tumors. Aromatic amines such as 2-naphthylamine and 4-aminobiphenyl, which is the first identified carcinogens resulting from dye industry exposures, causes bladder cancer. Aldehydes such as formaldehyde and acetaldehyde are commonly present in our daily life from smoking. Other carcinogens present in cigarette smoke are vinyl chloride, and ethylene oxide [12, 13].

Cigarette smoke also contains oxidants such as nitric oxide and free radicals that are involved in oxidative damage produced by cigarette smoke. Cigarette smoke contains diverse carcinogens. PAH, N-nitrosamines, aromatic amines, 1,3-butadiene, benzene, aldehydes, and ethylene oxide are among the most important carcinogenic compounds present in cigarette smoke [12].

3.2. Polycyclic aromatic hydrocarbons

Polycyclic aromatic hydrocarbons (PAHs) are a group of organic compounds composed of two or more fused aromatic (benzene) rings containing only carbon and hydrogen atoms. PAHs containing two and three rings are present in vapor phase in atmosphere as they have low molecular weight. However, PAHs with five rings or more are largely bound to particles and considered the most hazardous to humans. PAHs with intermediate molecular weight (four rings) are allocated between vapor and particulate phases. More than 11 carcinogenic PAHs were detected in the air of industrial countries. The most widely-spread PAHs compound is benzo[a]pyrene which is used as a marker for total exposure to carcinogenic PAHs.

Polycyclic hydrocarbons differ in their carcinogenicity; some have weak carcinogenic effect like, the compound dibenzo[a,c]anthracene, while others have potent carcinogenicity like 3-methylcholanthrene and 7,12-dimethylbenzo[a]anthracene [14].

PAHs are released into the environment form the combustion of carbon containing materials at high temperature. Indoor air contamination by PAHs occurs from indoor emission sources such as smoking, cooking, domestic heating with fuel stoves and open fireplaces, as well as from intrusion of outdoor air [14].

PAHs emissions from motor vehicle, power generation plants, waste incinerators and open burning are considered the main component of outdoor sources in industrialized countries. In developing countries, cooking and heating with solid fuels such as wood, agricultural residues or coal remains the main contributing source of indoor PAHs air pollution [14].

Individual exposure to PAHs occurs via inhalation of air, consumption of food and water, and dermal contact with soil and dust. Indoor air would be the major source contributing to the PAHs exposure through inhalation, as people spent 80–93% of their time indoors [14].

PAHs are easily absorbed from the gastrointestinal tract of human, as they are highly lipid soluble. Then they are rapidly distributed in a various tissues with a tendency for localization in fatty tissues. PAHs metabolized via the cytochrome P450s and epoxide hydrolase enzymes [14].

The carcinogenic potential of PAHs has been well established for decades, and evidence to date has resulted in many of these compounds being labeled as reasonably carcinogenic. Lung tumors have been detected in animals exposed to PAHs. In vitro studies showed that c-myc expression, adduct formation, and cell-cycle progression are altered in lung epithelial cells exposed to PAHs [15].

The mechanisms of carcinogenesis of PAHs have been extensively investigated. PAHs might cause DNA adducts. Recent studies indicate that PAHs can alter cell signaling cascades that control cell communication, growth, and immune functions. PAHs have been shown to act through nuclear receptors [15].

3.3. Nitrosamines

Nitrosamines are a class of approximately 300 compounds and about 90% of them have been found to be carcinogenic. For example dimethylnitrosamine causes liver cancer, whereas some of the tobacco specific nitrosamines cause lung cancer. Nitrates and nitrites occur naturally in fruit and vegetables, which are considered as an important part of a healthy diet in most countries. Nitrates and nitrites are often used as food additives in processed meats such as ham, bacon, sausages and hot dogs to prevent toxin production by Clostridium Botulinum (the microorganism responsible for botulism), and preserve meat products recognizable appearance and flavor as well [13].

Nitrosamines are produced by chemical reactions of nitrates or its reduced form nitrites with amines in the meat during its processing, storage, and cooking. N-nitrosodimethylamine

(NDMA) is one of the most frequently occurring nitrosamines in our dietary foods. NDMA is a potent carcinogen, associated with increased risk of malignant tumors of liver, lung, and stomach [13].

Nitrates (NO_3) and nitrites (NO_2) are inorganic compounds, composed of a single nitrogen atom (N) and a number of oxygen atoms (O). It is believed that nitrates themselves are relatively inert, and activated by nitrate reductase enzyme from bacteria in the mouth into to nitrites. Then nitrites are converted to nitrous acid by the acidic juices in stomach, which further reacts with amines to form nitrosamines. The carcinogenesis of nitrosamines could be through gene mutation and DNA adductions. A high consumption of processed meats was correlated to an increased gastric cancer risk, and many people consider nitrates/nitrites as the main reason for that [13].

3.4. Aflatoxins

Aflatoxin is a potent human carcinogen. It is a naturally occurring toxic metabolite produced by certain fungi (Aspergillus flavis). Aflatoxins are an interesting example of DNA damaging agents from a natural source. Among the aflatoxins of natural origin, aflatoxin B1 is the most potent hepatocarcinogen and considered to be the most toxic. Aflatoxins are regularly found in improperly stored staple commodities such as cassava, corn, cotton seed, millet, peanuts, rice, sesame seeds, and wheat [16].

Aflatoxins may be metabolized in the liver to a reactive epoxide intermediate or hydroxylated to become the less harmful aflatoxin M_1. Aflatoxins are commonly ingested through contaminated food. Animals fed contaminated food can pass aflatoxin transformation products into eggs, milk products, and meat. However the most toxic type of aflatoxin B_1, can permeate through the skin. It has been suggested that aflatoxins induce p53 gene mutations in hepatocytes [16].

3.5. Drugs and chemotherapy

Many drugs have carcinogenic potential such as intercalating antibiotics or nitroimidazole derivatives like metronidazole. The mechanism of action of nitroimidazoles is through reduction of the nitro group in predominantly anaerobic environments leads to formation of reactive intermediate products and hence destruction of DNA strands. Antimicrobial agents can be directly toxic, can interact with other drugs to increase their toxicity, or can alter microbial flora to cause infection by organisms that are normally saprophytic [17].

The majority of cytostatic agents (like: melphalan, nitrosourea, etoposide) are potentially carcinogenic. Certain tumors have been triggered by chemotherapy. Furthermore, some cytostatic agents have an immunosuppressive effect which renders the organism unable to eliminate mutated cells efficiently.

Owing to increased survival rates after chemotherapy, some patients develop years after primary therapy secondary malignancy. Most of secondary malignancies appear in the first 10 years after chemotherapy, especially after alkylating agents or nitrosourea derivatives. Of the alkylating agents, ALKERAN (melphalan), also known as L-phenylalanine mustard, phenylalanine mustard, LPAM, or L-sarcolysin, is a phenylalanine derivative of nitrogen mustard.

According to previous studies, alkylating agents such as cyclophosphamide, melphalan or procarbazine have the strongest leukemogenic potential [18].

3.6. Pesticides

Pesticides are a group of biologically active natural and synthetic chemicals, which are used to kill unwanted harmful insects, fungi, rodents and plants. All pesticides contain biologically active compounds that are purposely designed to interfere with normal biologic processes in target organisms. Therefore, individuals exposed to certain pesticides may be at risk to the development of certain cancers. Exposure to these pesticides could be through occupational exposures, the ingestion of contaminated food and water, by absorption through the skin, or by inhalation during application [19].

Currently, evidence supports that pesticides containing arsenic and ethylene oxide have the potential to cause cancer in humans. Pesticides may cause cancers by affecting cellular proliferation, apoptosis, and cell communication and inducing oxidative stress through non-genotoxic mechanisms. For example, 1,1,1-Trichloro-2,2-bis(*p*-chlorophenyl)-ethane (DDT) is one of the most well-known organochlorine carcinogenic pesticides. DDT tumorigenesis has been shown to be caused by tissue damage through oxidative mechanisms, alter cell signaling pathways (MAPK) that regulate growth, or activate the oncogene erb-B2 [20].

Though DDT was banned in the United State in the early 1970s, it is still used in other countries, and high levels of DDT has been detected in air, water, soil, plants, animals, and human tissues. The organochlorine pesticide 1,1,1-trichloro-2,2-bis (p-chlorophenyl)-ethane (DDT), is a well-known and widely dispersed "environmental estrogen" (World Health Organization Criteria no. 9; Geneva, Switzerland (1979)".

3.7. Arsenic

Inorganic arsenic has been suggested to be a human carcinogen since 1977. Arsenic is emitted into the atmosphere mainly from anthropogenic sources and a small amount from natural sources. Individuals may be exposed to arsenic compounds through contaminated food and drinking water or air emissions from industrial facilities that manufacture pesticides, glass, and cigarette tobacco [21].

Evidence suggests that there is a strong association between arsenic exposure and the development of skin, lung, bladder, kidney, liver, and colon cancers. The mechanism by which arsenic causes cancer is not well understood. It has been proposed that Arsenic does not interact with DNA, but indirectly causes chromosome aberrations, genomic instability, and aberrant DNA methylation in promoter regions of genes [22].

3.8. Dioxins

Dioxins are a group of structurally related compounds produced from industrial and combustion activities such as bleaching of paper, the manufacture of some pesticides, waste incineration, and fuels burning. They could be released from natural sources such as volcanic eruptions and forest fires. Dioxins are found in air, soil, water and food sources. Sufficient evidence from human epidemiologic and mechanistic studies showed an association between dioxins and various cancers including soft tissue sarcoma, lymphoma, leukemia, and Hodgkin disease. TCDD is the well-studied dioxin, which is known to be human carcinogen [23].

The mechanism responsible for dioxin-mediated carcinogenesis is via activation of the aryl hydrocarbon (Ah) receptor resulting in a wide spectrum of biologic responses, including altered metabolism, growth, and differentiation. It has been suggested that Dioxin alters multiple integrated cell signaling pathways, namely, the MAPK-ERK pathway through activation of tumor necrosis factor-alpha (TNF-a) and epidermal growth factor (EGF). Others suggested mutations in the proto-oncogene H-ras [24].

3.9. Asbestos

Asbestos is a group of six naturally occurring fibrous silicate minerals, namely: chrysotile, actinolite, amosite, anthophyllite, crocidolite, and tremolite. Chrysotile constitutes about 90% of the commercially used asbestos worldwide. Asbestos is released into the environment from natural and man-made sources and has been detected in air, soil, drinking water, food, and medicines. Asbestos toxicity occurs after a long latent period of about 15–40 year after initial fiber exposure. Occupational exposure to any type of asbestos increases the risk of lung cancer and mesothelioma [25].

More than 50 countries have banned the mining and/or use of all types of asbestos. However, past and current occupational asbestos exposures, and non-occupational domestic asbestos exposure originating from existing buildings that contain enormous amounts of the fibers and neighborhood exposures in communities living near asbestos mining, remains a global health challenge [26].

The carcinogenesis of asbestos is not fully understood. However, asbestos is a genotoxic agent that can induce direct DNA damage, gene transcription, and protein expression important in modulating cell proliferation, cell death, and inflammation [25].

Author details

Maher Soliman

Address all correspondence to: maher.soliman@daad-alumni.de

Oncology Department, Faculty of Medicine, Alexandria University, Alexandria, Egypt

References

[1] Torre LA, Bray F, Siegel RL, Ferlay J, Lortet-Tieulent J, Jemal A. Global cancer statistics, 2012. CA: A Cancer Journal for Clinicians. 2015;**65**(2):87-108

[2] Bray F, Moller B. Predicting the future burden of cancer. Nature Reviews. Cancer. 2006; **6**:63-74

[3] Pitot CH, Loeb DD. Fundamentals of Oncology. 4th ed. New York: Marcel Dekker; 2002. 41p

[4] Pott P. The Chirurgical Works of Percivall Pott, Vol. 5, Chirurgical Observations Relative to the Cataract, the Polypus of the Nose, the Cancer of the Scrotum, the Different Kinds of Ruptures, and the Mortification of the Toes and Feet. London: L. Hawes, W. Clarke and R. Collins; 1775

[5] Miller EC. Some current perspectives on chemical carcinogenesis in humans and experimental animals: Presidential address. Cancer Research. 1978;**38**:1479-1496

[6] Yamagawa K, Ichikawa K. Experimentelle Studie über die Pathogenese der Epithelialgeschwülste. Mitteilungen of Medical Faculty of Imperial University of Tokyo. 1915;**15**: 295-344

[7] "IARC Monographs". Monographs.iarc.fr. Retrieved 2017-10-5

[8] Gibbs WW. Untangling the roots of cancer. Scientific American. 2003;**289**(1):56-65

[9] Kling J. Put the blame on methylation. The Scientist. 2003;**16**(12):27-28

[10] Barrett JC, Shelby MD. Mechanisms of human carcinogens. Progress in Clinical and Biological Research. 1992;**374**:415-434

[11] Hecht SS. Tobacco smoke carcinogens and lung cancer. Journal of the National Cancer Institute. 1999;**91**:1194-1210

[12] Hecht SS. Etiology of cancer: Tobacco. In: TV DV, Lawrence ST, Rosenberg SA, editors. Devita, Hellman & Rosenberg's Cancer. Principles & Practice of Oncology. 8th ed. Philadelphia: Lippincott Williams & Wilkins; 2008. p. 148-165

[13] Oliver CP, Gloria MBA, Barbour JF, Scanlan RA. Nitrate, nitrite and volatile nitrosamines in whey-containing food products. Journal of Agricultural and Food Chemistry. 1995;**43**:967-969

[14] Air Quality Guidelines for Europe. 2nd ed. Copenhagen: WHO Regional Office for Europe; 2000 Polycyclic Aromatic Hydrocarbons. (WHO Regional Publications, European Series, No. 91)

[15] Menzie CA, Potocki BB, Santodonato J. Exposure to carcinogenic PAHs in the environment. Environmental Science and Technology. 1992;**26**:1278-1284

[16] McPherson M. Mycotoxin testing with aran gas: Aflatoxin B1 mycotoxin destruction using allotropic oxygen O4, O5, and O6. The Journal of Microbiology. 2015;**2**(6):00068

[17] Neu HC, Gootz TD. Medical Microbiology. 4th ed. University of Texas Medical Branch; Galveston; 1996. ISBN-10: 0-9631172-1-1

[18] Jones RB, Frank R, Mass T. Safe handling of chemotherapeutic agents: A report from the Mount Sinai Medical Center. CA: A Cancer Journal for Clinicians. 1983;**33**:258-263

[19] Alavanja MC, Samanic C, Dosemeci M, et al. Use of agricultural pesticides and prostate cancer risk in the agricultural health study cohort. American Journal of Epidemiology. 2003;**157**:800-814

[20] Bounias M. Etiological factors and mechanism involved in relationships between pesticide exposure and cancer. Journal of Environmental Biology. 2003;**24**:1-8

[21] Guo HR, Wang NS, Hu H, Monson RR. Cell type specificity of lung cancer associated with arsenic ingestion. Cancer Epidemiology, Biomarkers & Prevention. 2004;**13**:638-643

[22] Shi H, Shi X, Liu KJ. Oxidative mechanism of arsenic toxicity and carcinogenesis. Molecular and Cellular Biochemistry. 2004;**255**:67-78

[23] Bertazzi PA, Zocchetti C, Guercilena S, et al. Dioxin exposure and cancer risk: A 15-year mortality study after the "Seveso accident." Epidemiology. 1997;**8**:646-652

[24] Cole P, Trichopoulos D, Pastides H, Starr T, Mandel JS. Dioxin and cancer: A critical review. Regulatory Toxicology and Pharmacology. 2003;**38**:378-388

[25] MacDonald L. The health hazards of asbestos removal. JAMA. 1992;**267**:52-53

[26] Mossman BT, Bignon J, Corn M, Seaton A, Gee JB. Asbestos: Scientific developments and implications for public policy. Science. 1990;**247**:294-301

Chapter 5

What's New Among Cancer Etiology Horizon?

Trinanjan Basu

Additional information is available at the end of the chapter

http://dx.doi.org/10.5772/intechopen.71305

Abstract

The commonest saying goes as "cancer has no answer," we have really come a long way in that aspect. From being able to detect and diagnose the disease early, effective treatment modalities, improvement in therapeutic outcome and even effective palliative measures. The research focus emphasized upon detecting preventable risk factors. Tobacco a Global culprit is often discussed as the most important risk factor for cancer. Modern day life and with its so-called stress measures are the ones often been blamed without a concrete scientific evidences. Psychological makeup of a person, emotional stress and cellular phones are intricately associated with a modern lifestyle. In this chapter we would be focusing upon the causal relationship between these factors and malignancy with available scientific literature. At the end we would present possible measures to avoid them and any future research areas to be looked upon.

Keywords: cancer, emotional stress, psychological factors, cellular phones, modern lifestyle, habituation, modifiable risk factors

1. Introduction

Cancer is a term coined by the great Greek physician Hippocrates (460–370 BC). He is considered the "Father of Medicine." Hippocrates used the terms carcinos and carcinoma to describe non-ulcer forming and ulcer-forming tumors. Later on Galen (130–200 AD), another Roman physician used the term oncos (Greek for swelling) to describe tumors. Oncos is the root word for oncology or study of cancers.

It has been described in ancient mummies and over several years it has awakened a sense of fear and loss among the Human race. However technology also progressed at a rapid rate and main therapeutic modalities to treat cancer become a triad of surgery, chemotherapy and radiotherapy.

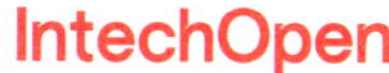

Parallel to these early diagnosis and preventive measures have also been researched in a large scale. This brings us to a domain called etiological factors for cancer. Tobacco has been linked to all head and neck cancers, esophageal cancers, bladder cancer especially, whereas dietary factors are predominant in breast and colon malignancies [1–5]. Interestingly few of the literature dates even more than 50 years back and current data also includes personal sexual behavior, Human papilloma virus infection (HPV) and tobacco in smokers as known risk factors.

These are often mentioned and often discussed issues. Effective strategies in cases of known risk factors have also been developed. Cancer vaccine is one such preventive step. In the case of cervical cancer a preventable vaccine is also been developed and shows promising outcome [6, 7].

Modern day lifestyle also brings along stress in terms if not only physical factors but also emotional issues. Low mood, depression and chronic anhedonia are household terns these days. There have been infrequent reports regarding emotional stress being causative factor for cancer [8–10]. Till date this is an important issue which lacks concrete evidence.

The other modern day risk being cellular phones aka mobile phones. Childhood brain tumors have been linked to it in several reports and it might have some significance. But again a large database and definite evidence is still to come out [11–13].

In this section we would elaborate the available literature related to these two less discussed etiologies of cancer viz. emotional/psychological stress and cellular phones. We would try and find if at all any link exists between them and related issues as per different sites of cancers.

2. Emotional stress

2.1. Introduction

Emotional stress, psychological factors or stressful life events these terms are often used interchangeably. Whatever may be the definition it has long been speculated to be linked to cancer development? The assumption of an association between stress and cancer is popular in the lay public [14]. Long back in 1992 Baghurst et al. described preventable issues but most of them were diet related. There was however a mention about environmental factors but emotional stress was not highlighted. Doll and Peto in 1985 also elaborate the dietary risk factors in different cancers and incidentally stress was highlighted to be a major contributory factor in colon, lung and breast cancers [15].

2.2. Definition

World Health Organization (WHO) defined health as "a state of complete physical, mental and social well-being and not merely the absence of disease or infirmity" [16]. With over half a decade and World witnessing several changes the WHO definition also should focus on the ability to adapt and self-manage in face of social, physical, and emotional challenges [17]. With the change in socio-cultural and demographic profile across world social support and emotional stress were linked to chronic diseases. As per American Psychosomatic Society social support is defined as "information leading the subject to believe that he is cared for and loved, esteemed, and a member of a network of mutual obligations [18]." The article enumerates that social support can protect people during crisis from a wide variety of pathological states like low birth weight to death, from arthritis through tuberculosis to depression, alcoholism, and the social breakdown syndrome. It has bigger implications like reduction in the amount of medication required, acceleration of recovery and compliance to medical regimens prescribed. These data never actually stated development of cancer related to social stress.

2.3. Pathophysiology

Psychological health itself is a difficult domain to assess. Aspects of psychological well-being like self-acceptance, positive relations with others, autonomy, environmental mastery, purpose in life and personal growth were mainly analyzed [19]. All these give a hint of link to chronic disorder and may be malignancy but without much evidence. Long back Evans suggested that the death of a spouse or other close relation could be an important cause of cancer. It was stated that "cancer is a miscarriage of this driving force, under the influence of the collective unconscious which is unrestrained after the patient has given up hope and interest in life (when the objective attachment is broken), that is, after the conscious has given up the struggle with the unconscious" [20]. However the study also could not establish a direct link. There is also no physiological mechanism to account for an increase in the incidence of or mortality from cancer after stressful events has yet to be specified in detail [8]. Loss of an important emotional relationship has been identified in several studies as an event with a high risk of subsequent illness [20–22]. Psychological stress activates the nervous system and the hypothalamic-pituitary-adrenal axis, leading to release of hormones such as glucocorticoids and norepinephrine. It has been shown that stress and the subsequent hormonal dysfunction can cause impairment of DNA repair and hence can suppress the immune system. Additionally, stress may lead to epigenetic silencing: altering DNA methylation and histone acetylation and all these are important in tumor development [23–25].

There is a separate discipline which studies these factors and called as psychoneuroimmunology. The multistep immune reactions are either inhibited or enhanced as a result of previous or parallel stress experiences, depending on the type and intensity of the stressor. As a rule both stressors and depression are associated with the decreased cytotoxic T-cell and natural-killer-cell activities. This further affect processes such as immune surveillance of tumors. This will lead to the events that modulate development and accumulation of somatic mutations and genomic instability [24].

From the time of the ancient Greeks, there has been an interest in the relationship between psychological states and cancer. Epidemiologic evidences have supported the role of biobehavioral risk factors in cancer progression. These are namely social adversity, depression, and stress. This is important both in initiation and progression phases [26, 27].

Early research on central nervous system (CNS) effects on cancer predominantly focused on the following:

a. Down-regulation of the immune response as a potential mediator of impaired surveillance for metastatic spread [27–31].

b. Stress effects on DNA repair [32, 33].

It is to be understood that there is no singular system available in explaining the biological effects of stress pathways on cancer progression. Over the last 10 years, the focus of mechanistic biobehavioral oncology research has broadened and it includes examination of the effects of stress on (a) tumor angiogenesis; (b) invasion and anoikis; (c) stromal cells in the tumor microenvironment, and (d) inflammation [27].

The salient features and how they affect immune system and cancer development or progression is enumerated in **Table 1**.

Biobehavioral factors	**Main cause**	**Pathophysiology**	**Implications**
Cellular immune response in cancer progression [34, 35]	Negative psychosocial states, such as chronic stress, depression, and social isolation	Down-regulation of the cellular immune response, mediated largely by adrenergic and glucocorticoid signaling	1. Depression has also been associated with a poorer cellular immune response to specific antigens in breast cancer 2. One study reported that depressed patients with hepatobiliary carcinoma had lower NK cell numbers and shorter survival compared to their non-depressed counterparts [36]
Angiogenesis and invasion [37–40].	Cancer-related mortality largely results from the spread of cancer cells from the primary tumor to other sites in the body, a process called metastasis. Successful metastatic spread requires several sequential steps, including angiogenesis, proliferation, invasion, embolization, and colonization of a new secondary site	Angiogenesis: this process is tightly controlled by a variety of positive and negative factors secreted by both tumor and host cells in the tumor microenvironment	Stress hormones such as norepinephrine (NE) have been shown to induce production of IL-6 and IL-8 by ovarian cancer and melanoma cells demonstrating effects of stress response pathways on tumor signaling mechanisms
Stress effects on anoikis [41–44]	Anoikis is the normal process of programmed cell death (apoptosis) occurring when anchorage-dependent cells become separated from the ECM. Cancer cells acquire the ability to resist anoikis, thus enhancing their ability to migrate, re-attach, and establish themselves in secondary sites	Catecholamines were found to protect ovarian cancer cells from anoikis, both in vitro and in vivo. These effects were mediated by focal adhesion kinase (FAK), a tyrosine kinase that promotes cell adhesion, which demonstrated increased activation (phosphorylation of pFAKY397) in response to NE. Clinically, elevated levels of pFAKY397 were observed in the tumor tissue of ovarian cancer patients reporting depression and those with higher levels of tumor NE	Ovarian cancer progression

Biobehavioral factors	Main cause	Pathophysiology	Implications
Stromal cells in the tumor microenvironment [43–46]	Tumor growth is to a large extent shaped and promoted or inhibited by signaling between tumor cells and the cells of the microenvironment. In addition to effects of stress hormones on tumor cells, there are marked effects on host cells such as macrophages in the tumor microenvironment	Monocytes are drawn to the tumor microenvironment by tumor-derived chemotactic factors and then differentiate into macrophages. However, under the influence of the pro-inflammatory microenvironment, macrophages are induced to shift from their phagocytic phenotype to a pro-tumor phenotype that produces tumor promoting factors such as VEGF and MMPs, while simultaneously down-regulating the cellular immune response by production of immunosuppressive cytokines such as IL-10 and TGFβ (75–78). TAMs are thus directly involved in promoting angiogenesis, tumor proliferation, invasion, metastases, and down-regulation of adaptive immunity. TAM infiltration is also associated with poorer survival	In ovarian cancer patients, biobehavioral risk factors that have been associated with higher NE levels, such as depression and stress
Glucocorticoid dynamics and cancer progression [47–49]		Glucocorticoids can directly mediate processes promoting tumor growth as well. Cortisol has been shown to stimulate growth of prostate cancer cells (85) and to enhance proliferation of human mammary cancer cells by nearly two-fold	In a murine breast cancer model, social isolation induced an elevated corticosterone stress response, greater tumor burden and alterations in gene expression in metabolic pathways that are known to contribute to increased tumor growth

Table 1. Stress and different pathophysiology.

2.4. Childhood cancers

It is altogether a different entity. Investigators have tried to assess the link between early life stress and development of childhood cancers. It is a unique scenario and in developed countries it is a leading cause of child deaths. Almost half of childhood cancers are diagnosed before 5 years of age and thus the importance of identifying early life risk factors for developing prevention strategies [50–53]. There is a certain physiological aspect also but like in adults the pathways are not very clear.

Large population-based cohort studies from Denmark and Sweden showed a small but statistically significant overall increased risk of childhood cancer was observed among children exposed to bereavement owing to the death of a family member. Exposure was also associated with CNS tumors and leukemia [53].

2.5. Conclusion

There is a definite correlation between stress and immunologic pathways for development of cancer and also for progression. In the clinical literature, lack of perceived social support is a factor that emerges repeatedly in associations with biological variables related to cancer progression, and social isolation has shown similar effects in the preclinical literature. Understanding what it is about social relationships that underlie these associations will be important in future research. Additional questions include the following: How much stress, in terms of thresholds or chronicity, is needed to modulate tumor-related pathways?

Many clinical studies even if prospective have failed to highlight life time stress as causative factor for cancer. The results of a large, prospective, population-based study therefore do not support the hypothesis that life stress, when defined as stressful life events, increases the risk for developing cancer [10].

3. Cellular phones

3.1. Introduction

There are three main reasons why people are concerned that cell phones (also known as "mobile" or "wireless" telephones) might have the potential to cause certain types of cancer or other health problems. Various literature reviews actually gives a very conflicting results. The exposure among pediatric and adult population is different and so as the outcome. As a potential etiology for cancer, cellular phones are yet to be regarded as common pathogens. As Munshi et al. describes "Centuries ago, we advanced from pigeons to postal services as a more modern means to communicate. Since then, communication has made quantum leaps, buoyed by the successes in physics and technology. From crude telephone sets to modern landline, cordless phones and finally cellular phones" [11].

3.2. Background knowledge

Mobile phones first came to use in the early 1990s for professional work-related reasons, and henceforth have attained tremendous growth, becoming able symbols for consumer status and needs. At present, nearly 5 billion people worldwide own cellular phones. India herself can boast of 800 million cellular phone users [54].

Another review by Munshi and Jalali highlighted how the fear of cellular phones and cancer develop. A decade ago a man in Florida, US sued a cell phone company alleging it lead to brain tumor in his wife [55]. The scientific evidence shows that mobile phones emit electromagnetic radiation (radiofrequency, RF) that is essentially non-ionizing. (frequencies between 300 MHz and 300 GHZ) [56–58]. The specific absorption rate (SAR) measures the energy dose that subjects exposed to RF absorb and is expressed in power (watts) by tissue mass (kilograms) [W/kg]. Effects of this dose deposition by use of cellular phones, however, take long to manifest. In some cases, this duration may be 10 years or more.

In general public there can be 3 reasons of concern:

a. Cell phones emit radiofrequency energy (radio waves), a form of non-ionizing radiation, from their antennas. Tissues nearest to the antenna can absorb this energy.

b. The number of cell phone users has increased rapidly. As of December 2014, there were more than 327.5 million cell phone subscribers in the United States, according to the Cellular Telecommunications and Internet Association. This is a nearly threefold increase from the 110 million users in 2000. Globally, the number of subscriptions is estimated by the International Telecommunications Union to be 5 billion.

c. Over time, the number of cell phone calls per day, the length of each call, and the amount of time people use cell phones have increased. However, improvements in cell phone technology have resulted in devices that have lower power outputs than earlier models [59].

It is to be noted that cell phones are often held tightly against the head. Electromagnetic radiation is governed by an interesting law known as the inverse square law. This essentially means that if we increase distance from the source by a factor of 2, the exposure gets reduced by 1/4th. It is for this reason, that distance from the device is a critical factor which decides the exposure received from a particular device. It is for the same reason that, if indeed a true risk exists, children would be at particular risk because their skulls are thinner. Also the cumulative lifetime exposure of children to cell phones would likely be greater than the exposure of current adults [11].

3.3. Clinical studies

Most of the work in cancer etiology and cellular phones has been based on brain tumors and parotid/salivary gland tumors because of the vicinity between these structures and cellular phone when used by an individual. Among brain tumors also most studies linked to glioma, meningioma and acoustic neuroma/schwannomas [11, 55].

There has been a meta-analysis published in JCO in 2009 about cellular phones and cancer risk. Myung et al. have selected initial 465 articles meeting their criteria and finally 23 case-control studies, which involved 37,916 participants were chosen. They found that a significant positive association (harmful effect) was observed in a random effects meta-analysis of eight studies using blinding, whereas a significant negative association (protective effect) was observed in a fixed-effects meta-analysis of 15 studies not using blinding. Mobile phone use of 10 years or longer was associated with a risk of tumors in 13 studies reporting this association (odds ratio = 1.18; 95% CI, 1.04–1.34) [60].

In reply to the above Stang et al. Criticized these random effects and have pointed out flaws related to the methodology. They have also highlighted their own data from uveal melanoma. After their initial case report they carried out case-control study on uveal melanoma focusing on mobile phone use and used the same detailed exposure assessment as the Interphone study used. The authors could not corroborate their previous results that showed an increased risk of uveal melanoma among regular mobile phone users. They accepted that probabilistic multiple error sensitivity analyses to evaluate the potential of exposure misclassification bias and selection bias did not explain the null result [61, 62].

The Interphone study group published the outcomes of an interview-based, case-control study with 2708 glioma and 2409 meningioma cases and matched controls. The study was conducted in 13 countries using a common protocol. The result of the study suggested that no increase in risk of glioma or meningioma was observed with use of mobile phones [63]. The cell phone companies faced these challenges and as of now they claim that Cell phone technology too is rapidly advancing and the electromagnetic exposure is progressively less with newer phones [64].

The World Health Organization (WHO) set up an expert panel to evaluate the effect of cell phones on the human body. On May 31, 2011 the expert panel said that cell phones might possibly cause side effects. The International Agency for research on Cancer (IARC) panel found cell phones to be "possibly carcinogenic," and stated that heavy cell phone use might or might not cause glioma [65]. Further in 2015 it was declared in a multicentric study that cell phone radiation can cause brain tumors and this to be categorized as probable human carcinogen category 2A. This study stated that previous IARC classification of Group 2B (possible) carcinogen in 2011 should be reclassified as a Group 2A (probable) carcinogen [12].

The basis of the above was another large scale epidemiologic study called CERENAT study which was a French case-control study of cases ≥16 years of age diagnosed between June 2004 and May 2006 included 253 glioma and 194 meningioma cases with two age- and gender-matched controls per case selected between 2005 and 2008. They included Potential confounders such as the level of education, smoking, alcohol consumption, and occupational exposures to pesticides, extremely low frequency electromagnetic fields (ELF-EMF), radiofrequency electromagnetic fields (RF-EMFs), and ionizing radiation. Risks of glioma were reported for heavy mobile phone use (≥896 cumulative hours of use). When heavy mobile phone use was examined by years since first use, glioma risk increased from >1 year since first use, to >2 years and to >5 years, OR 2.89, [95% confidence interval (CI) 1.41–5.93], OR 3.03, (95% CI 1.47–6.26), and OR 5.30, (95% CI 2.12–13.23), respectively. There was a borderline significant risk for glioma in the temporal lobe. This study also suggested risk for meningioma but lesser than glioma [66].

Interestingly these EM radiations can both initiate and promote tumor progression. In an Australian study of regional hospital-based data for the years 2000–2008, Dobes et al. stated, a significant increasing incidence in glioblastoma multiforme (GBM) was observed in the study period particularly after 2006 [67]. An increasing incidence of brain tumors during 2003–2012, 41.2% among men and 46.1% in women has been noted in Denmark, cases of GBM nearly doubled in the previous 10 years [68].

3.4. Precautions

Munshi and Jalali have beautifully highlighted how we can take few precautions. (1) Use the cell phone whenever it is really needed. For most routine work and casual talks, use the regular landline connection. (2) Discourage children from excessive use of cell phones.

(3) Whenever possible, use a wired ear piece connected to the cell phone. (4) Avoid cell phone use when the signal is weak. (5) Consider alternating between left and right ear while talking on cell phone. (6) Use texting (SMS) instead of calling when possible [55]. Morgan et al. also stated that until further evidence is available, it is prudent to follow the ALARA standard used in pediatric radiology. The ALARA approach would require hardware and software designers to create proximity sensors and embed flash notices regarding simple advisories about safer use within devices [12].

3.5. Conclusion

The data regarding cellular phone usage and cancer risk is ever emerging. We have some progress towards stronger association as IARC classification changed. As time advances newer and more mature results will come up. At the same time it is also true that a billionaire cellular phone Industry will also come up with safer devices. We will also need prospective data as the major limitation of epidemiological studies addressing the health effects of mobile phone use is related to exposure assessment. These limitations are inherent in case-control studies [69]. Borrowing the lines from Munshi et al. "it may be some time before we know if the friendly gizmos in our hands have the ability to cause aggressive tumors, for the time being, you have the free choice—to talk or not to talk" [11].

Acknowledgements

This was a unique opportunity. I would like to thank my parents (Mrs. Karabi Basu and Mr. PM Basu) for always supporting and not forcing me in all my decisions and my wife (Reshmi Ghosh) who has been my friend, philosopher, counselor and motivator. I always draw inspiration from daily patients in my practice and several thoughts have actually originated from their sufferings. I would take this opportunity to thank my MD guide Prof. Anup Majumdar, my teachers at Tata Memorial Hospital, Mumbai (Dr. Siddhartha Laskar, Dr. Sarbani G Laskar, Dr. JP Agarwal and all other teachers and friends). A personal thank you to my seniors Dr. Shikha Goyal, Dr. Deepak Gupta and Dr. Susovan Banerjee who always encouraged me to perform better, and to my childhood friend Dr. Shirshendu Sinha, a practicing psychiatrist at Mayo College, USA, for believing in me. Last but never the least, thank you for everything to the Almighty.

Author details

Trinanjan Basu

Address all correspondence to: trinanjan.doctor@gmail.com

HCG Apex Cancer Centre, Borivali West, Mumbai, India

References

[1] Armstrong B, Doll R. Environmental factors and cancer incidence and mortality in different countries, with special reference to dietary practices. International Journal of Cancer. 1975;**15**:617-631

[2] Wynder EL, Bross IJ, Feldman RM. A study of the etiological factors in cancer of the mouth. Cancer. 1957;**10**:1300-1323

[3] Wynder EL, Bross IJ. A study of etiological factors in cancer of the esophagus. Cancer. 1961;**14**:389-413

[4] Gandhi AK, Kumar P, Bhandari M, Devnani B, Rath GK. Burden of preventable cancers in India: Time to strike the cancer epidemic. Journal of the Egyptian National Cancer Institute. 2017;**29**:11-18

[5] Shah A, Malik A, Garg A, Mair M, Nair S, Chaturvedi P. Oral sex and human papilloma virus-related head and neck squamous cell cancer: A review of the literature. Postgraduate Medical Journal. 2017 Aug 4 pii: postgradmedj-2016-134603

[6] Jindal HA, Kaur A, Murugan S. Human Papilloma Virus vaccine for low and middle income countries: A step too soon? Human Vaccines & Immunotherapeutics. 2017 Aug 28:1-3. DOI: 10.1080/21645515.2017.1358837 [Epub ahead of print]

[7] Huh WK, Joura EA, Giuliano AR, Iversen OE, de Andrade RP, Ault KA. Final efficacy, immunogenicity, and safety analyses of a nine-valent human papillomavirus vaccine in women aged 16-26 years: A randomised, double-blind trial. Lancet. 2017 Sep 5. pii: S0140-6736(17)31821-4. DOI: 10.1016/S0140-6736(17)31821-4 [Epub ahead of print]

[8] Jones DR, Goldblatt PO, Leon DA. Bereavement and cancer: Some data on deaths of spouses from the longitudinal study of Office of Population Censuses and Surveys. British Medical Journal (Clinical Research Ed.). 1984;**289**:461-464

[9] Taylor C, Trowbridge P, Chilvers C. Stress and cancer surveys: Attitudes of participants in a case-control study. Journal of Epidemiology and Community Health. 1991;**45**:317-320

[10] Bergelt C, Prescott E, Grønbaek M, Koch U, Johansen C. Stressful life events and cancer risk. British Journal of Cancer. 2006;**95**:1579-1581

[11] Munshi A. Cellular phones: To talk or not to talk. Journal of Cancer Research and Therapeutics. 2011;**7**:476-477

[12] Morgan LL, Miller AB, Sasco A, Davis DL. Mobile phone radiation causes brain tumors and should be classified as a probable human carcinogen (2A) (review). International Journal of Oncology. 2015;**46**:1865-1871

[13] McKinney PA. Brain tumours: Incidence, survival, and aetiology. Journal of Neurology, Neurosurgery, and Psychiatry. 2004;**75**(Suppl 2):ii12-17

[14] Baghurst KI, Baghurst PA, Record SJ. Public perceptions of the role of dietary and other environmental factors in cancer causation or prevention. Journal of Epidemiology and Community Health. 1992;**46**:120-126

[15] Doll R, Peto R. The causes of cancer: Quantitative estimates of avoidable risk of cancer in the United States today. Journal of the National Cancer Institute. 1981;**66**:1193-1265

[16] Callahan D. The WHO definition of 'health'. Studies—Hastings Center. 1973;**1**:77-88

[17] Nobile M. The WHO definition of health: A critical reading. Medicine and Law. 2014; **33**:33-40

[18] Cobb S. Presidential Address-1976. Social support as a moderator of life stress. Psychosomatic Medicine. 1976;**38**:300-314

[19] Ryff CD. Happiness is everything, or is it? Explorations on the meaning of psychological well-being. Journal of Personality and Social Psychology. 1989;**57**:1069-1081

[20] Evans E. A Psychological Study of Cancer. New York: Dodd Mead and Co; 1926

[21] LeShan L. An emotional life history pattern associated with neoplastic disease. Annals of the New York Academy of Sciences. 1966;**125**:780-793

[22] Muslin HL, Gyarfas K, Pieper WJ. Separation experience and cancer of the breast. Annals of the New York Academy of Sciences. 1966;**125**:802-806

[23] Kiecolt-Glaser JK, Glaser R, Williger D, et al. Psychosocial enhancement of immunocompetence in a geriatric population. Health Psychology. 1985;**4**:25-41

[24] Reiche EM, Nunes SO, Morimoto HK. Stress, depression, the immune system, and cancer. The Lancet Oncology. 2004;**5**:617-625

[25] Hunter RG. Epigenetic effects of stress and corticosteroids in the brain. Frontiers in Cellular Neuroscience. 2012;**6**:18

[26] Brock AJ. Greek Medicine: Being Extracts Illustrative of Medical Writers from Hippocrates to Galen. London, England: JM Dent and Sons; 1929

[27] Lutgendorf SK, Sood AK. Biobehavioral factors and cancer progression: Physiological pathways and mechanisms. Psychosomatic Medicine. 2011;**73**:724-730

[28] Levy S, Herberman R, Lee J, Whiteside T, Kirkwood J, McFeeley S. Estrogen receptor concentration and social factors as predictors of natural killer cell activity in early-stage breast cancer patients. Natural Immunity and Cell Growth Regulation. 1990;**9**:313-324

[29] Levy S, Herberman R, Lippman M, D'Angelo T, Lee J. Immunological and psychosocial predictors of disease recurrence in patients with early-stage breast cancer. Behavioral Medicine. 1991;**17**:67-75

[30] Levy S, Herberman R, Maluish A, Schlein B, Lippman M. Prognostic risk assessment in primary breast cancer by behavioral and immunological parameters. Health Psychology. 1985;**4**:99-113

[31] Levy SM, McCabe PM, Schneiderman N, Field TM, Skyler JS, editors. Stress, Coping and Disease: Behavioral and Immunological Host Factors in Cancer Risk. Hillsdale, NJ: Lawrence Erlbaum Associates; 1991. p. 237-253

[32] Glaser R, Thorn B, Tarr K, Kiecolt-Glaser J, D'Ambrosio S. Effects of stress on methy-transferase synthesis: An important DNA repair enzyme. Health Psychology. 1985;**4**:403-412

[33] Kiecolt-Glaser JK, Stephens RE, Lipetz PD, Speicher CE, Glaser R. Distress and DNA repair in human lymphocytes. Journal of Behavioral Medicine. 1985;**8**:311

[34] Blomberg BB, Alvarez JP, Diaz A, Romero MG, Lechner SC, Carver CS, Holley H, Antoni MH. Psychosocial adaptation and cellular immunity in breast cancer patients in the weeks after surgery: An exploratory study. Journal of Psychosomatic Research. 2009;**67**:369-376

[35] Sephton SE, Dhabhar FS, Keuroghlian AS, Giese-Davis J, McEwen BS, Ionan AC, Spiegel D. Depression, cortisol, and suppressed cell-mediated immunity in metastatic breast cancer. Brain, Behavior, and Immunity. 2009;**23**:1148-1155

[36] JL GDA, Gamblin TC, Olek MC, Carr BI. Depression, immunity, and survival in patients with hepatobiliary carcinoma. Journal of Clinical Oncology. 2007;**25**:2397-2405

[37] Fidler IJ. The pathogenesis of cancer metastasis: The 'seed and soil' hypothesis revisited. Nature Reviews. Cancer. 2003;**3**:453-458

[38] Folkman J. What is the evidence that tumors are angiogenesis dependant? Journal of the National Cancer Institute. 1990;**82**:4-6

[39] Folkman J, Klagsbrun M. Angiogenic factors. Science. 1987;**235**:442-447

[40] Senger DR, Galli SJ, Dvorak AM, Perruzzi CA, Harvey VS, Dvorak HF. Tumor cells secrete a vascular permeability factor that promotes accumulation of ascites fluid. Science. 1983; **219**:983-985

[41] Shanmugathasan M, Jothy S. Apoptosis, anoikis and their relevance to the pathobiology of colon cancer. Pathol Int. Apr 2000;**50**(4):273-279

[42] Yawata A, Adachi M, Okuda H, et al. Prolonged cell survival enhances peritoneal dissemination of gastric cancer cells. Oncogene. 1998;**16**:2681-2686

[43] Pollard JW. Tumour-educated macrophages promote tumour progression and metastasis. Nature Reviews. Cancer. 2004;**4**:71-78

[44] Sica A, Allavena P, Mantovani A. Cancer related inflammation: The macrophage connection. Cancer Letters. 2008;**267**:204-215

[45] Sica A, Rubino L, Mancino A, et al. Targeting tumour-associated macrophages. Expert Opinion on Therapeutic Targets. 2007;**11**:1219-1229

[46] Sica A, Schioppa T, Mantovani A, Allavena P. Tumour-associated macrophages are a distinct M2 polarised population promoting tumour. European Journal of Cancer. 2006;**42**:717-727

[47] Zhao XY, Malloy PJ, Krishnan AV, et al. Glucocorticoids can promote androgen-independent growth of prostate cancer cells through a mutated androgen receptor. Nature Medicine. 2000;**6**:703-706

[48] Simon WE, Albrecht M, Trams G, Dietel M, Holzel F. In vitro growth promotion of human mammary carcinoma cells by steroid hormones, tamoxifen, and prolactin. Journal of the National Cancer Institute. 1984;**73**:313-321

[49] Elenkov IJ. Glucocorticoids and the Th1/Th2 balance. Annals of the New York Academy of Sciences. 2004;**1024**:138-146

[50] Anderson LM. Environmental genotoxicants/carcinogens and childhood cancer: Bridgeable gaps in scientific knowledge. Mutation Research. 2006;**608**:136-156

[51] Kaatsch P. Epidemiology of childhood cancer. Cancer Treatment Reviews. 2010;**36**:277-285

[52] Parkin DM, Whelan S, Ferlay J, et al. Cancer Incidence in Five Continents VIII. Vol. 155. Lyon, France: IARC Scientific Publications (IARC); 2002

[53] Momen NC, Olsen J, Gissler M, Cnattingius S, Li J. Early life bereavement and childhood cancer: A nationwide follow-up study in two countries. BMJ Open. 2013;**3**(5):e002864. DOI: 10.1136/bmjopen-2013-002864

[54] Hoskote SS, Kapdi M, Joshi SR. An epidemiological review of mobile telephones and cancer. The Journal of the Association of Physicians of India. 2008;**56**:980-984

[55] Munshi A, Jalali R. Cellular phones and their hazards: The current evidence. National Medical Journal of India. 2002;**15**:275-277

[56] Heynick LN, Johnston SA, Mason PA. Radio frequency electromagnetic fields: Cancer, mutagenesis, and genotoxicity. Bioelectromagnetics. 2003;**6**:S74-100

[57] Chang SK, Choi JS, Gil HW, Yang JO, Lee EY, Jeon YS, et al. Genotoxicity evaluation of electromagnetic fields generated by 835-MHz mobile phone frequency band. European Journal of Cancer Prevention. 2005;**14**:175-179

[58] Hardell L, Sage C. Biological effects from electromagnetic field exposure and public exposure standards. Biomedicine & Pharmacotherapy. 2008;**62**:104-109

[59] Available from: https://www.cancer.gov/about-cancer/causes-prevention/risk/radiation/cell-phones-fact-sheet. [Accessed: May 2017]

[60] Myung SK, Ju W, McDonnell DD, Lee YJ, Kazinets G, Cheng CT, et al. Mobile phone use and risk of tumors: A meta-analysis. Journal of Clinical Oncology. 2009;**27**:5565-5572

[61] Stang A, Anastassiou G, Ahrens W, et al. The possible role of radiofrequency radiation in the development of uveal melanoma. Epidemiology. 2001;**12**:7-12

[62] Stang A, Schmidt-Pokrzywniak A, Lash TL, et al. Mobile phone use and risk of uveal melanoma: Results of the risk factors for uveal melanoma case-control study. Journal of the National Cancer Institute. 2009;**101**:120-123

[63] Interphone Study Group. Brain tumour risk in relation to mobile telephone use: Results of the INTERPHONE international case-control study. International Journal of Epidemiology. 2010;**39**:675-694

[64] Pope L, Silva P, Almeyda R. Phone applications for the modern day otolaryngologist. Clinical Otolaryngology. 2010;**35**:350-354

[65] Available from: http://www.iarc.fr/en/media-centre/pr/2011/pdfs/pr208_E.pdf [Accessed: 2011 Aug 2]

[66] Coureau G, Bouvier G, Lebailly P, et al. Mobile phone use and brain tumours in the CERENAT case-control study. Occupational and Environmental Medicine. 2014;**71**:514-522

[67] Dobes M, Khurana VG, Shadbolt B, Jain S, Smith SF ea. Increasing incidence of glioblastoma multiforme and meningioma, and decreasing incidence of Schwannoma (2000-2008): Findings of a multicenter Australian study. Surgical Neurology International. 2011;**2**:176

[68] The Danish Cancer Society. The Increase in New Cases of Aggressive Brain Cancer. http://www.cancer.dk/Nyheder/nyhedsartikler/2012kv4/Kraftigstigningihjernesvulster.html. [Accessed: 22-09-2014]

[69] Auvinen A, Toivo T, Tokola K. Epidemiological risk assessment of mobile phones and cancer: Where can we improve? European Journal of Cancer Prevention. 2006;**15**:516-523